PRAIS

"I would hi̦
non-traditiona̦ ......v.c. ι̇ ι̇s original and
insightful. The students would love it."
—JUDY BATTAGLIA

"The text is well organized and up to date.
Photovoice is clearly explained as it relates to data
collection."
—STACEY CALLAWAY

"Photovoice for Social Justice *is an excellent
resource for both students and practitioners who are
interested in using research to empower underserved
communities through action and advocacy. Anyone
who is interested in social justice research will find
it useful.*"
—EMMANUEL CLOTTEY

"This text is basic enough for those who are
being introduced to photovoice—and qualitative
methods—for the first time, yet comprehensive
enough to guide the experienced researcher in
developing and implementing a photovoice
project."
—TAMARA J. LYNN

"The method is strong, [including] participatory
engagement with groups, developing an open
dialogue amongst groups that have similar issues
and those that don't offer learning experiences for
facilitator and people in each group."
—MICHELE WASHINGTON

Photovoice for Social Justice

Visual Representation in Action

We dedicate this book to our teacher, colleague and friend, Dr. Kathleen M. Roe, who taught us the critical importance of humility and passion for community work. Her commitment to making the world a better place is unparalleled, and without her, this book truly would not have been written.

Photovoice for Social Justice

Visual Representation in Action

Jean M. Breny
Southern Connecticut State University

Shannon L. McMorrow
Western Michigan University

Los Angeles | London | New Delhi
Singapore | Washington DC | Melbourne

QUALITATIVE RESEARCH METHODS SERIES

Series Editor: David L. Morgan, *Portland State University*

The *Qualitative Research Methods Series* currently consists of 58 volumes that address essential aspects of using qualitative methods across social and behavioral sciences. These widely used books provide valuable resources for a broad range of scholars, researchers, teachers, students, and community-based researchers.

The series publishes volumes that:

- Address topics of current interest to the field of qualitative research.

- Provide practical guidance and assistance with collecting and analyzing qualitative data.

- Highlight essential issues in qualitative research, including strategies to address those issues.

- Add new voices to the field of qualitative research.

A key characteristic of the Qualitative Research Methods Series is an emphasis on both a *"why"* and a *"how-to"* perspective, so that readers will understand the purposes and motivations behind a method, as well as the practical and technical aspects of using that method. These relatively short and inexpensive books rely on a cross-disciplinary approach, and they typically include examples from practice; tables, boxes, and figures; discussion questions; application activities; and further reading sources.

New and forthcoming volumes in the Series include:

Qualitative Instrument Design: A Guide for the Novice Researcher
Felice D. Billups

How to Write a Phenomenological Dissertation
Katarzyna Peoples

Reflexive Narrative: Self-Inquiry Towards Self-Realization and Its Performance
Christopher Johns

Hybrid Ethnography: Online, Offline, and In Between
Liz Przybylski

Doing Systematic Fieldwork through Cognitive Ethnography

For information on how to submit a proposal for the Series, please contact:

- David L. Morgan, Series Editor: morgand@pdx.edu
- Leah Fargotstein, Acquisitions Editor, SAGE: leah.fargotstein@sagepub.com

FOR INFORMATION :

SAGE Publications, Inc.
2455 Teller Road
Thousand Oaks, California 91320
E-mail: order@sagepub.com

SAGE Publications Ltd.
1 Oliver's Yard
55 City Road
London, EC1Y 1SP
United Kingdom

SAGE Publications India Pvt. Ltd.
B 1/I 1 Mohan Cooperative Industrial Area
Mathura Road, New Delhi 110 044
India

SAGE Publications Asia-Pacific Pte. Ltd.
18 Cross Street #10-10/11/12
China Square Central
Singapore 048423

Printed in the United States of America

This book is printed on acid-free paper.

ISBN: 9781544355474

Library of Congress Control Number: 2020948984

Acquisitions Editor: Leah Fargotstein

Editorial Assistant: Natalie Elliott

Production Editor: Astha Jaiswal

Copy Editor: diacriTech

Typesetter: diacriTech

Proofreader: Lawrence W. Baker

Indexer: diacriTech

Cover Designer: Dally Verghese

Marketing Manager: Victoria Velasquez

20 21 22 23 24 10 9 8 7 6 5 4 3 2 1

Brief Contents

Detailed Contents

Preface

WHY THIS BOOK?

Photovoice is a research method that transcends academic disciplines. It can be an essential tool for both academics and community practitioners to uncover action areas for social justice by prioritizing the world views and stories of community members from their own lens and in their own words. This book, *Photovoice for Social Justice: Visual Representation in Action*, will detail and illustrate the community-based participatory research method of photovoice, a method ideal for understanding and facilitating action to eliminate social inequities. The major underpinning of photovoice is that it is a participatory research method, one that utilizes feminist theory, Freirian approaches, and a constructivist paradigm towards research. What this means is that it is an ideal method for uncovering the lived experiences among communities and people who may not otherwise have a voice in traditional (positivist) research methods and approaches. Not only is it participatory, but it is a way to facilitate expression of aspects of participants' lives in ways that go beyond words and numbers, by bringing in visual day-to-day experiences.

THE GOAL OF THIS BOOK

Photovoice (a) considers the research participants as co-researchers (the participatory part) and (b) has the purpose of translating the results into action of some kind, such as advocacy, policy change, or a health promotion program. The point of view, then, is that a participatory method like photovoice that both engages participants as co-researchers and captures lived experiences, is the ideal way to uncover precursors to social and cultural inequities. Thus, the overarching goal of this book is to provide practical, concrete steps for conducting photovoice as practice-based research with results to translate into programs or policies designed to eliminate inequities and increase social justice.

THE AUDIENCE FOR THIS BOOK

Diverse and multidisciplinary academics and community practitioners across the social, health, and educational sciences will benefit from this book. It could be used as a core text in any class that focuses primarily on photovoice methodology specifically, or participatory and qualitative research methods in general. Photovoice is an excellent tool for the practice of public health and other applied disciplines that incorporate conducting community assessments and formative research, so the book would make an excellent supplementary text for courses focused on program planning and other applied methods of community-based work.

THE FEATURES OF THIS BOOK

A special feature of this book is that our original scholarship is utilized as case illustrations in almost every chapter. We felt it important to share these examples as a way to help readers understand the method, including challenges and lessons we have learned through experience. Other examples from the vast photovoice literature were also carefully selected to share experiences of researchers using photovoice across a range of disciplines. The variety and expanse of the populations of focus, social and health issues of interest, and findings from the work currently being done are rich and important.

This book is organized to follow a typical research project process and begins, first, with Chapter 1 introducing readers to the method and theoretical underpinnings of photovoice. Chapter 2 covers important and unique ethical considerations as well as aspects of working with an institutional review board for approvals to do a photovoice research project. Chapters 3, 4, and 5 cover the step-by-step process of planning and conducting a photovoice research project including steps to prepare, recruitment of participants, managing photovoice focus group discussions, and collecting and analyzing data. Chapter 6 concludes the book with observations about and a brief introduction to current and future iterations of other visually based qualitative research methods like videovoice and digital storytelling.

Acknowledgments

We gratefully acknowledge the participants/co-researchers we have had the privilege of working with and learning from over the years. We hold dear their trust in us as they shared their stories, fears, passions, and hopes for a socially just world. SAGE and the authors would like to thank the reviewers of this manuscript:

Allissa V. Richardson, University of Southern California

Andrea Romero, University of Arizona

Beth Powers, Millersville University of Pennsylvania

Carl Siebert, Boise State University

Denise Blum Oklahoma State University

Emmanuel N. Clottey, Louisiana State University Shreveport

Judy Battaglia, Loyola Marymount University

Karyn Madore, JSI Research and Training Institute, Inc.

Michele Y. Washington, Fashion Institute of Technology

Stacey L. Callaway, Rowan College of South

Tamara J. Lynn, Fort Hays State University

About the Authors

Jean M. Breny is a professor and department chair of the Department of Public Health at Southern Connecticut State University. Since 1994, she has worked in community-based health promotion practice and research in a variety of practice and academic settings. Her research and scholarship aim to eliminate health disparities through an antiracist lens, using photovoice and qualitative methods, that inform public health practice and advocacy. Her work has been recognized internationally as Dr. Breny was an invited speaker to the First International Symposium of Health Promotion and Communications in Istanbul, Turkey, and she was a Fulbright Senior Scholar in Izmir, Turkey. Dr. Breny also holds a visiting professorship at the Public Health Institute at Liverpool John Moores University and is an associate scientist at the Center for Interdisciplinary Research on AIDS (at Yale University). She is a past president of the Society for Public Health Education (SOPHE).

Shannon L. McMorrow is an assistant professor in the School of Interdisciplinary Health Programs at Western Michigan University. Since 1998, she has worked in community-based public health as a practitioner and academic in multiple U.S. states, Belize, and Uganda. Her research and writing projects seek to illuminate important, underemphasized social and cultural aspects of public health issues in order to eliminate health inequities. She prioritizes the use of community-based participatory research approaches, with a predominant focus on using photovoice. She has published and presented her photovoice work locally, nationally, and internationally in diverse and multidisciplinary venues such as the Great Lakes Chapter of the Society for Public Health Education, the European International Studies Association, *Health Education & Behavior*, and the *Journal of International Migration and Integration*.

Introduction

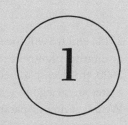

A photo exhibit in a local government center shows photographs of a community in disarray. Evidence of safety issues, violence, and no place to exercise. The mayor gets the message that a community center that once was thriving in this community, must be rebuilt.

A group of transgender women stand proudly next to their photos showing the triumphs of their transitions, their stories of strength in an otherwise transphobic society. The greater community sees the importance of their visibility, the need to be inclusive to transgender people.

PURPOSE OF THIS BOOK

In this book, *Photovoice for Social Justice*, we detail and illustrate the method's ideal use for understanding and eliminating health and social inequities and promoting social justice. The practical foundation and the scholarly purpose of our book is to guide social justice researchers and practitioners on the use of photovoice. Research methods that deeply explore community member's lived experiences with how they are treated by society are ideal in addressing social inequalities. Qualitative methods, in particular, are most useful in this (Patton,

2015) and we will focus on a step-by-step process of how to conduct qualitative, photovoice studies. As we write this book in the spring of 2020, the deeply rooted social and racial inequities across the United States are being brought to light to the general public as never before. We are seeing disparate, unjust outcomes from COVID-19 and the long-overdue uprising in reaction to ongoing police brutality and unjust murder primarily targeting Black people. It is our hope and intent that this book serve as a tool for a wide array of professionals to confidently move forward in using photovoice as one method in the renewed fight for racial and social justice for all.

HISTORY AND BACKGROUND OF PHOTOVOICE

If it is true that "a picture is worth a thousand words," then photovoice is a method beyond comparison. The mileage we get from photos illustrating the lived experiences of people goes beyond numbers and data typically used in health and social research. When accompanied by the dialogue and words of people who participate in photovoice, the method produces data with potential for use as a powerful advocacy tool to promote social justice.

The major underpinning of photovoice is that it is a participatory research method, one that utilizes feminist theory, Freirean approaches, and a constructivist paradigm toward research (Wang & Burris, 1994, 1997; Wang, Burris, & Ping, 1996). What this means is photovoice is an ideal method for uncovering the lived experiences among communities and people who may not otherwise have a voice in traditional (positivist) research methods and approaches. Not only is photovoice participatory, but also it is a way to have people express aspects of their lives in ways that go beyond words and numbers, by bringing in visual day-to-day experiences.

Photovoice as a participatory action-oriented research method: (a) considers the research participants as co-researchers (the participatory part) and (b) has as its purpose translating the results into action, such as a new or revised policy or a health promotion program (Wang & Burris, 1997). The point of view, then, is that a participatory method like photovoice that redefines research participants as *co-researchers* as well as captures their lived experience is the ideal way to uncover what the precursors are to social and cultural inequities. With the information gleaned from photovoice, action-oriented and community-based researchers can translate the results into programs or policies that will help eliminate inequities to increase social justice. Photovoice may or may not uncover new information during the course of a project; however, its critical contribution is that it offers new perspectives and ways of understanding community issues directly from communities or populations.

At the time of writing this book, a quick literature search reveals nearly 3,800 journal articles mentioning photovoice have been published across journals from a multitude of disciplines including political science, youth services, social work, education, international development, and public health. This includes photovoice studies uncovering and illustrating all kinds of issues related to health and social justice (Breny & Lombardi, 2017; Carnahan, 2006; Castleden, Garvin, & First Nation, 2008; Findholt, Michael, & Davis, 2011; Genoe & Dupuis, 2013; Keller, Fleury, Perez, Ainsworth, & Vaughan, 2008; Madden & Breny, 2016; Mamary, McCright, & Roe, 2007; Martin, Garcia, & Leipert, 2010; McMorrow & Saksena, 2017; McMorrow & Smith, 2016; Strack, Magill, & McDonagh, 2004; Wang & Burris, 1997; Wang et al., 1996). The list of social experiences that could potentially be explored using photovoice is seemingly endless and includes critical topics facing society today such as racial injustice, violence, homelessness, healthcare access, education, experiences of sex workers, experiences of refugees and other immigrants, and more.

Theoretical Underpinnings of Photovoice

Drs. Caroline Wang and Marianne Burris are often noted as the pioneers of the method we now call photovoice. Their groundbreaking work occurred in the context of international development work with Chinese migrant women and brought a new era of using photography and the visual image as research data (Wang et al., 1996). The method as they conceptualized it is rooted in three theoretical foundations: (a) documentary photography, (b) Paulo Freire's theory and practice of critical consciousness and empowerment education (Freire, 1970), and (c) feminist theory. Understanding these conceptual frameworks is important for users of photovoice to grasp the great potential of the method to give voice to those who traditionally have not been heard.

Documentary Photography

The power of documentary photography is that it shows history and experiences through visual means. However, the power and ownership of the photographs remain with the photographer, despite who is being photographed. Photovoice, on the other hand, seeks to rebalance power to the photographer/research participants, hence putting "cameras directly into the hands of people who otherwise would not have access, and allows them to be recorders and potential catalysts, in their own communities" (Wang & Burris, 1994, p. 174). In this way, the research participants are photographers, interpreters, and participants all combined into one.[1]

Empowerment Education

Paulo Freire was a Brazilian educator and philosopher with lived experience of poverty and hunger that deeply informed his teaching methods. He utilized problem-based pedagogy, which involved learning through dialogue between farmworkers facilitated through using pictures as triggers for conversation starters (also called codes). These codes and subsequent dialogue not only helped the farmworkers learn Portuguese but also increased their personal empowerment. Through dialogues about farm life, they realized their place in society and that there was room for change—resulting in their critical awareness or consciousness of their ability to make change (Freire, 1970). "The pedagogy is problem-based and contextual: the knowledge that results is practical and directed towards action" (Wang & Burris, 1997, p. 172). This critical consciousness is the ideal aim of photovoice to achieve through putting co-researchers in control of what, when, and how they choose to take photos and also through dialoguing with pictures through a focus group style discussion.

---

[1] In this book, we refrain from using the term *subject* and will refer to people working in photovoice projects as either *research participants* or *co-researchers*.

Feminist Theory and Research

Feminist approaches to research and epistemology are similar to Freirean approaches to education in that they are intended to facilitate critical consciousness, to empower the research participants, and to aim to change policy. "As empowerment education has challenged traditional approaches to schooling, so have feminist critiques of positivist research methods and the construction of knowledge pushed new aims and methods of inquiry" (Wang & Burris, 1997, p. 175). One of the many ways that photovoice actualizes a feminist approach is through what Campbell and Wasco (2000) referred to as "reducing hierarchical relationships." Though a hierarchy exists with photovoice and there are still power imbalances between the researcher and the participants, the method explicitly seeks to reduce and minimize this hierarchy.

In sum, these three approaches/underlying theoretical concepts of documentary photography, empowerment education, and feminist theory are the basis of the photovoice method. They drive us to uncover the many truths in people's lived experiences: truths that need to be told by communities and heard by policymakers, change agents, and others in power—indeed, truths that are often best shown through visual means and with a goal of critical consciousness and change.

PHOTOVOICE FOR SOCIAL JUSTICE

Social justice is often applied as a vague and undefined term as many academics and practitioners committed to social justice tend to assume that others know what it means. Consequently, there are a variety of definitions that change slightly depending on the profession or academic discipline that is asked to define social justice. Therefore, for the purpose of this book, it is important to have a common, working definition. We love the definition offered by the Arcus Center for Social Justice Leadership (2020), which is:

> Social justice recognizes the inherent dignity of all people and valuing every life equally. Social justice calls for both personal reflection and social change to ensure that each of us has the right and the opportunity to thrive in our communities,

regardless of our identities. Those who strive for social justice believe in the triumph of our shared humanity.

Using this definition and considering the aforementioned description of photovoice, we can see that photovoice is inherently a method that lends itself as a tool for working toward social justice.

Photovoice is considered a community-based participatory research (CBPR) method, which means it is grounded in the philosophy that working collaboratively with communities on research as opposed to the traditional researcher-led approach results in steps needed for action (Minkler & Wallerstein, 2008). CBPR has been defined as:

> *A **collaborative** approach to research that **equitably** involves all partners in the research process and recognizes the unique strengths that each brings. CBPR begins with a research topic of importance to the community and has the aim of combining knowledge with action and **achieving social change**.* ... (Israel, Schulz, Parker, & Becker, 1998)

Thus, when researchers and practitioners choose photovoice as a method and commit to authentic engagement through CBPR, there is additional potential for social justice outcomes related to the *process* of engaging in photovoice. For example, a photovoice project can intentionally build skills such as photography, organization, and communication that empower participants as part of the implementation process of the study and contribute, at least in part, to the ability of participants to lead change in the community.

The three original goals of photovoice as articulated by Wang and Burris (1997) also link to social justice. They are to: (a) enable people to record and reflect their community's strengths and concerns, (b) promote critical dialogue and knowledge about important issues through large and small group discussion of photographs, and (c) reach policymakers (Wang & Burris, 1997). Although not all photovoice projects reach the stage of engaging policymakers, this is an important goal to keep in mind as an ultimate means of impacting social justice. For example, if a photovoice project engages people who are homeless in a particular city and their stories are shared with the local city council, then this may result in a city policy change that leads to more equitable economic or mental health treatment opportunities for the project population.

CONCLUSION

Photovoice is a research method that transcends academic disciplines. It can be an essential tool for both academics and community practitioners to uncover action areas for social justice by prioritizing the worldviews and stories of community members from their own lens and in their own words. In Chapter 2, we turn toward the first steps of planning for a photovoice study. This includes ethical considerations, an overview of institutional review boards (IRB), unique considerations for navigating an IRB with a photovoice study, and a case study for enhanced understanding of the concepts we cover in Chapter 2.

Ethical Issues and Navigating Institutional Review Boards

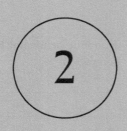

CHAPTER OVERVIEW

The aim of this chapter is to assist you with recognizing unique ethical considerations for photovoice and with planning accordingly for the application to the Institutional Review Board (IRB) at your institution. Photovoice can be a unique experience for researchers and participants and as noted in Chapter 1, photovoice has the potential to empower participants. However, along with that potential, there are distinct ethical considerations to recognize when using the photovoice method. These considerations are always important but may be even more so if you are using photovoice with marginalized, traditionally underrepresented, or oppressed populations. This chapter will discuss key ethical considerations from our experiences implementing photovoice studies as well as those noted previously by other researchers using photovoice from multiple disciplines. Simultaneously, we offer potential tips for addressing the ethical concerns that may assist with navigating IRB approval of studies using photovoice. Finally, we close this chapter with a case study illustrating our experience with navigating one IRB.

IRB EXPLAINED

A deep dive into all of the nuances of IRBs is beyond the scope of this book, but it is important to have a basic understanding of what an IRB is and how it works. An IRB is an administrative committee within your college or university that is established for the purpose of reviewing all research to ensure human subjects are protected and that the research methods are ethical. Most photovoice projects need to be approved by an IRB because the overarching intent is usually to share the results broadly beyond the classroom for advocacy. You will need to submit an application and wait for official approval from the IRB before starting your photovoice research. There are often modifications requested by the IRB, so it is best to plan ahead and submit the IRB application at least 6 months prior to the date you hope to start implementing your project. The forms, committee composition, timeline, and general processes vary a lot from institution to institution, so your first step is to investigate the process and requirements at your college or university. Most colleges and universities offer IRB materials online.

We advise students to seek guidance and mentorship from a faculty member with IRB experience if you are new to the process. Sometimes, the IRB may require a faculty member to serve as an investigator on your application, so it is best to determine whether your institution requires this and plan accordingly. There are different levels of review ranging from an expedited review involving only one or two reviewers and less time to a full board review involving all members of the committee meeting to discuss your proposal. Some populations, such as minor children under age 18, pregnant women, and people in prison, automatically lead to a full board review, so again, it is best to investigate the expectations and timelines at your institution to guide your planning process.

ETHICAL CONSIDERATIONS WITH PHOTOVOICE

Photovoice projects are often designed with social justice in mind as an outcome and a desire to tip the balance of power for marginalized populations, people who often have less of a voice due to structural inequities in society. Therefore, it is critical to recognize that the researcher or research team leading a photovoice project has the ethical responsibility for ensuring autonomy throughout the duration of the project. Simply defined, autonomy in research means that a participant makes their own decisions about what they will and will not agree to related to participation in a research study (Owonikoko, 2013). Additional ethical considerations for implementing photovoice covered in this chapter are informed consent, safety and privacy of co-researchers, the safety and privacy of people captured in photographs, and incentives and payments for participants. One critical point is that even though an IRB may approve your study, there is still an array of additional ethical considerations for you to acknowledge and potentially put into practice due to the nature of photovoice as a CBPR method aiming to reduce the inherent power imbalances present in most research.

CONSIDERATION FOR SPECIAL POPULATIONS

It is important to consider for a moment the use of photovoice in special populations such as people with different physical abilities, who are homeless, youth, or people with different developmental abilities. At first glance, photovoice seems to be a method limited to those who have the physical and intellectual ability to take pictures, meet in physical groups to discuss, and make decisions around how to best use the photos for social change. In fact, the beauty of a method like photovoice is that it is inherently adaptable and flexible enough to be tailored to fit any populations' needs, reading level, language ability, physical ability, geographic location, etc. Indeed, photovoice studies have been done within a spectrum of populations at differing levels of ability, such as people who are homeless (Seitz & Strack, 2016) and persons with physical disabilities (Dassah, Aldersey, & Norman, 2017). In all cases, you, as the project leader, can adapt photovoice to cater to the specific levels of capacity to ensure successful projects. For example, adaptations might include having someone else take photos for people who were physically unable to (LaDonna, Ghavanini, & Venance, 2015) or reducing, lengthening, or having one–one meetings about the photos taken (Bukowski & Buetow, 2011; Hodgetts, Radley, Chamberlain, & Hodgetts, 2007), recruiting through agencies that directly work with and serve these populations (Bredesen & Stevens, 2013), or selecting types of cameras that can accommodate physical disabilities (Greer, Hermanns, & Cooper, 2015).

The takeaway message here, one that we reiterate throughout this book, is that every photovoice project will be different and can be adapted to what will best serve the population of focus, the abilities and availabilities of the co-researchers, the research topic being explored, and the time and resources available to the research team. In sum, photovoice researchers do what needs to be done in order to facilitate a successful project leading to social change.

Informed Consent in Photovoice

There are different ways to ensure the autonomy of your participants in photovoice. The first, which is also required by all IRBs, is to design an informed consent process that is simple and clear. This includes directly stating the purpose of the project, benefits for participants or lack thereof, potential risks to participants, and that it is entirely their choice to participate in the project. This sounds deceivingly simple. One challenge may be balancing your IRB's requirements for written elements for informed consent with the desire to have simple language that will resonate with your participants. Sometimes, IRBs may require certain language in the informed consent form or process that leads to a lengthy document filled with technical jargon that may be above the reading level of your participants. If that occurs, then one suggestion is to advocate for your participants and negotiate a compromise that is acceptable for both you and the IRB. For example, you may be required to include all of the specific statements from the IRB in the informed consent form, but perhaps you can request to edit them to a simpler language that fits a reading level more closely aligned with the population with whom you are conducting your project.

With the informed consent process, another possibility may be to request IRB approval to conduct an oral informed consent as opposed to written if this seems like the best fit for the participants (Gordon, 2000). Another important way to promote autonomy for your participants is to engage in ongoing informed consent through the implementation of the entire project, which views informed consent as a dynamic process as opposed to a one-time occurrence at the beginning of a study (Kadam, 2017). Ongoing informed consent usually does not involve gathering signatures or official consent in the same way as the initial informed consent. Instead, you simply build a process into every photovoice session or meeting with participants in which you start out by reminding them that participation is optional and that they may decide not to participate in the project at any time that day or during the future. A sample of an informed consent form for photovoice is included in the Tools at the end of this chapter.

Safety of Participants

Safety is an important issue inherent to photovoice that you need to consider and build into both study implementation and the IRB application. In this context, safety should be considered broadly and comprehensively to include physical, psychological, and emotional safety. For some populations, it may be beneficial for the research team to have understanding and training in how to utilize a trauma-informed approach (Harris & Fallot, 2001).

One unlikely, but potential, risk to participants is from people who observe the photovoice study co-researchers taking photos, are uncertain what they are doing, feel threatened, and react with verbal or physical harm. A common way to address this is to dedicate at least one session to "Ethics and Safety" during your photovoice project that occurs prior to the study participants going out to take photos. Organization and approaches to this session vary widely, but the overarching goal is to explicitly address all ethical and potential safety concerns for the participants themselves in the context of the specific photovoice project and to detail concrete action steps that participants can take to protect their safety.

Our approach to ensure the safety of participants is to communicate unequivocally that their safety is an absolute top priority and there is not any photo or portion of the photovoice project that is more important than safety. For example, they may be in a situation where they see an opportunity to take a photo that they feel is an excellent representation of the aims of the project, but it involves community members engaging in illegal activities. In that case, we let participants know that taking the photo is not worth the risk. Another way we have handled this is to use guest speakers from the community who are familiar and respected by the participants. For example, for a project in a school with youth under 18, we invited a school resource/law enforcement officer who reiterated messages about safety and spoke frankly about specific risks to avoid during photovoice in that community. The approach will vary widely, but the key is to have a comprehensive plan to minimize safety risks in your photovoice project and to be prepared to provide details of your plan to the IRB.

Privacy of Research Participants

Protecting the privacy of people who participate in a research study is an ethical obligation for all researchers. It is important for you, as the person in charge of the photovoice study, to honestly communicate the risks to privacy with participation in a photovoice project. The nature of photovoice is such that it is nearly impossible for a participant to remain anonymous. For example, participants may end up taking "selfies," which means their face is in the photo. Even if the participants do not end up physically in the photographs that they take, their photos will often have identifiers such as parts of their home, school, community, or property that might allow someone looking at the photo to guess who they are. This may be of high concern for uniquely vulnerable populations needing anonymity such as those experiencing domestic violence, so it is certainly something to intentionally plan and address depending on the privacy needs of the specific population with whom you are working.

An additional area of privacy unique to photovoice is the protection of the privacy of people who are in the photos taken by the participants/co-researchers. There are a few different options that can be used. A common practice is to train participants to use a Photo Release Form, which means the participants talk with the people in their photos to explain the purpose of the project and have them give consent for their image to be shared in the photos by signing a form. There is one example in the Tools section at the end of this chapter. Participants first engage with potential photography subjects before taking their photo, explain the purpose of the study, ask if the person is willing to be in a photo, and obtain their signature. An additional benefit of this approach is that it also mitigates safety risks and enables you to be certain that the photos can be freely used and shared for purposes such as advocacy, presentations, or publications. The potential downsides are that it detracts from spontaneity and some people may refuse to be included. Another variation of this approach is to train participants to implement the Photo Release Form and obtain consent to share the photo *after* the photo has been taken and the participant has identified that this is an important photo for inclusion in the project and they'd like to share it in group discussions or more widely. A third possibility for protecting privacy of people in the photos of your participants is to have a concrete plan for fully blurring facial features or other identifying characteristics in photos. The benefit of this approach is retaining spontaneity and the ideal to have candid photos, whereas the downside is that the risk for identification of people, even with blurring photos, cannot be eliminated. In sum, there is always a possibility that people will be included in the photos, so the burden is on you as the researcher to have a clear, concrete plan to protect the privacy of people appearing in photographs for research.

Social media such as Facebook, Instagram, or Twitter is yet another area of importance to consider for protecting the privacy of participants. Chapter 6 delves a bit more into social media, but the overarching concern in the context of privacy protection is to make sure that you have an explicit plan for how social media will be handled in relation to your photovoice project. It may be that you decide not to use social media due to privacy concerns. In that case, you would want to communicate that with participants as a ground rule of the project or perhaps put it into writing to ensure that one participant does not violate the privacy of another participant by sharing photos of them or sharing photos that they took during the course of the photovoice project.

Incentives/Payment for Participants as Co-researchers

A final ethical issue to consider is the use of incentives for photovoice participants. Researchers from a wide variety of disciplines use incentives for a variety of reasons when implementing research. However, it is important to recognize that there is a diverse array of opinions about using incentives. One common ethical concern for conducting community-based research in partnership with community-based organizations is the potential for researchers setting an expectation or standard within the community that cannot be maintained by the organization after the researchers have completed the project. For example, one of our studies was conducted in partnership with a refugee resettlement agency that was well known across all groups of refugees in the city (McMorrow & Saksena, 2017; Saksena & McMorrow, 2017). When we proposed to offer photovoice participants financial incentives for participation in the project, there was reasonable and legitimate concern from the agency that the perception in the community might be that the incentive was coming from them and would be expected for participation in programs they offered. One way to manage this is to ensure that all stakeholders recognize the view of "participants as co-researchers" in photovoice. Then, to communicate that as such, there is an ethical obligation to remunerate them for the substantial time and work involved with attending photovoice training sessions, taking photos, attending photovoice discussion sessions, and potentially advocating for policy change. Yet again, the keys here are to have a definitive plan with a solid rationale and to be prepared to spell out the details in the IRB application. A literature review section of your IRB application that includes examples of prior use of incentives in photovoice may be a good tool to support your request.

NAVIGATING IRBs WITH A PHOTOVOICE STUDY

Navigating the IRB is closely aligned with the aforementioned ethical concerns. This is something that all researchers who work with human subjects need to do before beginning participant recruitment and photovoice is no exception. All photovoice projects will need approval from your university's IRB before implementation. A sample of the methods section of an IRB proposal is included in the Tools at the end of this chapter for you to get a general sense of the level of detail that is needed. Additionally, if you are working with a community agency, then you will need to find out if they have their own IRB and potentially follow their requirements as well. Students leading photovoice projects are often enabled by their faculty mentors to write the IRB application but usually need a faculty member to serve as the principal investigator for the study. In the same way that no photovoice project is exactly the same as another, IRBs vary vastly from institution to institution. They usually consist of a diverse range of university faculty representatives and often include community representatives as well. In some cases, the leader of an IRB aims to have a diverse representation of faculty who have a firm grasp of both quantitative and qualitative research methodology. In other cases, the IRB may have a disproportionate number of representatives who have limited knowledge of qualitative research and, sometimes, bias against qualitative methods. Similarly, there can be a diversity of familiarity and value for the photovoice method among potential IRB members reviewing the study.

We have collectively navigated five different IRBs and our experiences range from conducting education and advocacy for the importance of the method with one IRB who was not at all familiar with the method to a straightforward experience of securing approval quickly (Breny & Lombardi, 2017; Madden & Breny, 2016; McMorrow & Saksena, 2017; McMorrow & Smith, 2016; Ruff, Smoyer, & Breny, 2019). The overarching recommendation is to be prepared by thinking through all of the considerations listed in this chapter and accounting for them in your IRB application as well as be prepared to educate IRB members and advocate for the use of the method. It won't always be necessary, but preparation will ensure that you are ready to secure IRB approval and move on to the next step of implementing your study.

CASE ILLUSTRATION: AN IRB EXPERIENCE WITH A PHOTOVOICE PROJECT WITH MINORS

For this particular case, the photovoice study population was Black teenage girls between the ages of 13 and 17 who attended high school in an urban neighborhood with a high crime rate. All research involving minors require that parents give consent for participation in the research study and permission is obtained from the youth themselves, which is called assent. Obtaining assent from youth is an additional factor to consider if you are working with minors and a sample assent form is included in the Tools section at the end of this chapter. An important ethical concern for both the researcher and the IRB was ensuring participants were assenting to participate in the project. Additional considerations were obtaining their parents' informed consent, safety, and privacy of other minors in the school.

The university of the photovoice project researcher was a relatively small school with a historical focus on teaching and a less robust history of diverse research by faculty. Therefore, this necessitated education and advocacy for the photovoice method. For example, the first IRB submission was returned to the researcher with a long list of questions and modifications. The researcher met with the chair of the IRB to describe the method, advocate for the importance of using it, and seek advice from the chair on how to improve the application to address the particular concerns of that IRB. To address safety explicitly within the context of the environment of the study population, it was agreed that the school resource officer (police officer) would serve as a guest speaker for the photovoice training to focus on risks related to the neighborhood.

In terms of the concern about privacy of other minors in the school, the eventual compromise was that no photos of other people could be included in any public sharing of photos that emerged as data in the study. In retrospect, this is not a compromise that we would advise. Instead, if you find yourself in a similar scenario, we recommend continued advocacy to confirm that privacy could be ensured by blurring of people in photos or obtaining photo consent. One way to do this is to provide recent examples from the literature of other researchers who have utilized similar methods to address ethical concerns when using photovoice.

CONCLUSION

As with any research project, it is critical to build time into the planning of the project to think through the ethical considerations and potential risks to participants. The goal is to prepare for success right up front with concrete plans and backup plans. Photovoice projects introduce an additional layer of ethical concerns, beyond many traditional research approaches, due in part to the nature of the use of photography and the potential for a breach of anonymity. This chapter provided an example of how to navigate IRB boards to ensure protection of both research participants and research team members as well as samples of several tools that might be used. In the next chapter, we turn toward the next phase of getting your photovoice project started with concrete steps and tools to guide you through that process.

Chapter 2 Tools

1. Sample of IRB Application Methods Section for Photovoice Project

2. Sample Photovoice Photo-Release Approval Form: Investigating Social and Environmental Cues for Relationship Power: Photovoice Photo-Release Approval Form

3. Sample Consent Form for Participation in Photovoice Research: Exploring Young Men's Perceptions of Safer Sex Responsibility: Consent Form for Participation in Photovoice Research

4. Sample Youth Assent Form

Sample of IRB Application Methods Section for Photovoice Project

METHODS

There will be two groups: males and females. Participants will attend a total of four group sessions. Initially, they will receive a structured training program consisting of one 2-hour session of experiential skill building. The introductory session will include an Introduction to Photovoice and Principles of Documentary Photography (including ethics, informed consent, and communication skills). Following the initial training, participants will be asked to use their personal cameras or camera phones to take photo assignments.

Participants will be given a workshop on the ethics of camera use by the principal investigator. The ethics orientation will be conducted prior to the signing of informed consent forms. The purpose of this session is to ground participants in the responsibilities, power, ethics, and potential risks of taking pictures in the community. The group discussion in this session will include questions such as: What is an acceptable way to approach someone to take his or her picture? Should someone take pictures of other people without their knowledge? To whom might you wish to give photographs and what might be the implications? When would you not want to have your picture taken? (Wang & Burris, 1997). The youth will be instructed that photographs that do not have photo-release forms signed will not be displayed with the project. In addition, youth will be instructed to not take pictures of any illegal acts or nudity in their community and that any such photographs will be destroyed.

There will be four photo assignments with a follow-up discussion on each one. An initial question for the first photo assignment might be, "For people your age, what do relationships look like or mean?" Participants will then meet every 2 weeks for three additional sessions. At each session, the discussion will focus on the following questions, which comprise the SHOWeD technique: What do you See here?

What is really Happening here? How does this relate to Our lives? Why does this situation, concern, or strength exist? What can we Do about it? Themes will be identified and short descriptive pieces written. Other questions for photo assignments might include:

1. What messages do young girls receive about relationships?

2. How do men gain power in relationships?

3. What messages should be developed and targeted to young women to help them own their power?

Results of the photos and discussions will be structured around (a) identifying the cultural, environmental, and social messages that create an imbalance in power and (b) initiating discussions about gender imbalances and potential solutions.

Release forms will be used by participants when taking pictures of other people (See the following page).

Sample Photovoice Photo-Release Approval Form: Investigating Social and Environmental Cues for Relationship Power

PHOTOVOICE PHOTO-RELEASE APPROVAL FORM

Hi, my name is _____*\<insert your name\>*_____ and I am with Southern CT State University. I am involved in a Photovoice research project, where students from Southern are taking photographs of messages in the community that represent gender roles, can perpetuate gender roles in relationships, and also show relationship power. The photographs will be used to create discussions about youth and our community. The project is led by Dr. Jean Breny at Southern Connecticut State University (SCSU).

The photographs I take will be used for research and education purposes only, including use at lectures, conferences, and with published materials. No photographs that identify your family, other individuals, or me will be released without the written consent of those photographed.

I need your approval to use any photographs with you in them. If you agree, I need your signature on this photo-release form.

Please sign here: _____

Date: _____

Sample Consent Form for Participation in Photovoice Research: Exploring Young Men's Perceptions of Safer Sex Responsibility

CONSENT FORM FOR PARTICIPATION IN PHOTOVOICE RESEARCH

DR. JEAN M. BRENY, PRINCIPAL INVESTIGATOR

You are being asked to participate in a photovoice project. This project is being conducted as part of a research project on the social, cultural, and environmental factors that influence relationship power in 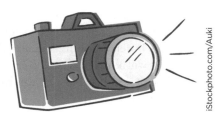heterosexual relationships. The principal investigator is Dr. Jean Breny in the Department of Public Health at SCSU. Please feel free to call Jean, at 203-XXX-XXXX, if you ever have any questions about this study or your involvement in this study. Alternatively, you can contact the SCSU HRPP at 203-XXX-XXXX. The project is funded through a grant from the Connecticut State University system.

The purpose of this photovoice project is to provide an in-depth and reflective look at how young people receive messages about gender norms from society and how they are translated into power imbalances in relationships. The research will enable participants to express their experiences through picture taking, dialogue, and conversation.

Your involvement will consist of attending a series of four focus group discussions to process and discuss pictures taken by you and others between these group sessions. With your permission, the group discussions will be tape-recorded for analysis purposes. These tape

istockphoto.com/Auki

recordings will be used to transcribe the focus groups and the transcripts read for themes in the analysis process. Your name, and any other identifying feature, will not appear on the transcript. At each group meeting, you will be given a photo assignment to be completed for the next session. These assignments will be decided upon by the group members and will focus on some aspect of relationship power and decision making. You will attend one introductory session on photovoice and receive your first photo assignment. We will all meet again in 2 weeks, where we will discuss that assignment and give you another one. This will continue until we have had four discussions. You will be given a gift card to the campus bookstore for your involvement in this project. It is expected that the project will be done within 4–5 weeks.

Your participation in this research project is completely voluntary and you can refuse to answer any question or you can leave before the end of the duration of the project. If you decide not to answer some questions or leave, your decision will not affect your relationship with the University or the researcher in any way.

Every effort is being taken to protect your identity. However, there is no guarantee that the information cannot be obtained by legal process or court order. You will not be identified in any report of this study and the only people who will be here today are you, other participants, the researcher, and an assistant. You can choose to use a fake name, and your real name will not be written down anywhere. Each focus group will be taped so that it can be transcribed. You can refuse this or can have the tape turned off at any time. If you agree to be tape-recorded, your name will not be on the transcription and the tape will be destroyed immediately after it has been transcribed. All data will be kept in a locked file cabinet and destroyed after 3 years.

The benefits of participation and talking about your experiences about relationship power will help this researcher, and others, develop relevant and effective STD/HIV prevention programs for people of your age. The only risk to you in participating in this group might be that you feel anxious talking about something personal and the time you spend here may take you away from other activities.

By signing below, you agree to participate in today's focus group.

_____   _____

Signature   Date

Sample Youth Assent Form

Project Title: Saginaw Valley State University Assessment of Barriers and Assets to Healthy Eating Using Photovoice by Youth in Saginaw, MI

Principal Investigator: _____

Community Partners: _____

Participant's Name: _____

In this research project, you and other participants are invited to take pictures and tell stories about the positive and negative influences on healthy eating in your life and community. This is a chance for you to teach others about what affects healthy eating in your life.

If you decide to take part in the project, you will be asked to:

- Take part in training and learn about taking photographs.

- Take pictures of things that influence healthy eating in your life and community.

- Meet with other participants to discuss each other's photographs. As part of the project, some discussion sessions may be audio- or video-taped and notes will be taken. You may also be asked to participate in an interview.

If you agree to participate, you will be assigned a disposable camera for taking pictures during the project. The project staff will develop the film. You will be given a copy of your developed pictures. By signing this consent form, you are agreeing to let the project staff use the photographs you take. Your name will never be used other than during discussions unless you wish to use your name or a pseudo-name.

At any time, you may ask us not to use any specific photograph(s) or story. If you wish to participate in the project and do not want our photographs or stories used, you may do so. You may also withdraw from the project at any time and there will be no negative consequences.

This research project is being conducted on behalf of Saginaw Valley State University in conjunction with the Saginaw High School Based Health Center operated by Health Delivery, Inc. If you have any questions about this project, you or your parent or guardian may contact Shannon McMorrow, Principal Investigator from Saginaw Valley State University xxx-xxx-xxxx or smcmorro@svsu.edu at any time. You may also contact the Chair, SVSU Human Subjects Institutional Review Board (xxx-xxx-xxxx or irbchair@svsu.edu) if you have any questions or problems that come up during the study.

Remember, your participation is completely voluntary. Signing this paper means that you have read this and that you want to be in the project. This is your decision. You may decline to participate in the project at any time.

This consent document has been approved for use for 1 year by the Human Subjects Institutional Review Board (HSIRB) as indicated by the stamped date and reference number in the upper right-hand corner. Subjects should not sign this document if the corner does not show a stamped date and reference number.

_____   _____
Print Your Name Here   Date of Birth

_____   _____
Sign Your Name Here   Today's Date

Getting Started With Your Photovoice Study

3

CHAPTER OVERVIEW

In this chapter, we turn to the nuts and bolts of initiating a photovoice project. As with any research study, photovoice projects usually begin with research questions or aims. Additionally, a starting point for some photovoice projects is a population of interest. Particularly when using photovoice as a means toward social justice, the population is often a group that may be considered marginalized or disempowered within the context where you are studying or researching. For example, in the cultural context of the United States, youth are a common population in photovoice projects because societal policies, systems, and norms lead to them having less of a voice than adults. Research question development for a photovoice study is similar to the general approach to research question development for other qualitative research but also contains unique considerations in terms of asking questions that can be best answered by photovoice.

Once you formulate a research question, it may need to be "translated" into language that is tailored for participants to understand what they are being asked to photograph—more about that in just a bit. Moving on to another major step to getting started, we cannot overstate the need for formulation of a project management plan because photovoice implementation requires a high level of preplanning and organization to maximize the quality of your project. After that, recruitment occurs with its own set of important considerations. Finally, a focus on technology choices and uses is crucial when getting started with a photovoice project. This chapter will dive into more detail for each of those important issues.

RESEARCH QUESTION, POPULATION, OR BOTH?

Sometimes photovoice studies that are initiated by researchers start with a population of focus, particularly if the researcher prioritizes promoting social justice and empowering participants. In these cases, there may not yet be a specific research question that you start out with. Instead, there may be a more general research question related to examining and uncovering the perspectives and experiences of that particular population in a particular setting through photovoice. An example of a broad set of questions in this instance might be, "What are the experiences of Black youth living in Kalamazoo, MI? What do they perceive as positives in their community and what do they perceive as negatives?" Other times, photovoice studies start with a more specific question of interest to the researcher. Photovoice has been used to address a staggering range of topics across the health and social sciences, such as, health, gender identity, discrimination, education, immigration, and migration. With this example, an iteration of the question into something more specific might be "What are the experiences of discrimination among Black youth living in Kalamazoo?" As you can see, the possibilities for photovoice questions are relatively endless. However, the questions must be open-ended instead of closed and should enable co-researchers to explore many facets of the topic being researched. If you go the route of starting a project with a research question, then we strongly recommend talking it over with the participants once you get to that stage of implementation and being open to iteration and change.

Other photovoice studies may be initiated by the participants/co-researchers. For example, in a university setting, college students may learn about the photovoice method in the classroom and decide it seems like an exciting tool to explore and advocate for an issue of importance on campus. In this example, it could be *issue* driven for the entire student population, such as lack of recycling and other environmental health services; or it could be *population* driven, such as international students wanting to explore the social and cultural experiences of international students on the campus. Either way, the students might then approach a faculty member to support them through the process, but the question and population have already been formulated by the co-researchers.

Yet another variation that we alluded to earlier is to engage in an iterative process to collaborate together with participants to develop more specific research questions and the photovoice mission. This may occur when the starting point is a population of interest and the researcher is open to the question evolving after the start of implementation. This also may occur if the researcher has a question in mind that revolves around a topic that can be open to interpretation and narrowing to more specificity by the participants themselves. For example, the researcher may set out with a specific question asking, "What are the experiences of immigrant women in the workplace in a particular city?," but then plan for the first couple of photovoice meetings to collaborate with participants to prioritize a more specific part of the workplace experience such as health, social support, or discrimination.

Another tactic that we have used with success in the past is to use a participatory approach with a partner agency to develop questions or choose study populations that are of interest in an applied nature. For example, one of our studies involved the first step of engaging a refugee resettlement agency to tell them about the photovoice method and inquire if it may be useful to inform their provision of services. From there, the agency identified a specific population they felt it would be useful to have more information about via a photovoice study. More details about this approach are detailed in the case illustration at the end of this chapter.

A crucial outgrowth of development of your research question(s) is thinking through how you will explain or "translate" questions to participants. Sometimes, you may be able to use the same or very similar language with your participants. For example, for the aforementioned example about experiences with discrimination for Black youth, you might say, "Take photos of your experiences with discrimination in Kalamazoo." However, other times, it may be necessary to fully translate your research questions into different, more accessible language for the population you are working with. For example, a research question in academic jargon for one of our studies was, "What are perceptions of Black teen girls about things that impact obesity in their environments?," which was translated to a photo mission of "Take photos of things in your home, school, and community that you think prevent obesity or lead to obesity" (McMorrow & Smith, 2016). It may also be an option to develop the "translation" in a participatory manner with the co-researchers by first sharing an academic version and then working together to see how the participants understand it and reformulate it in their own words.

Overall, as you can see, there are many ways to develop questions and/or start with a population as you work within the unique context and circumstances of your photovoice project. Whichever path you choose, recognize that developing research questions and the corresponding photo missions for photovoice is much like it is for other qualitative studies; it is a winding path with a multitude of different considerations that takes dedicated time (Miles, Huberman, & Saldana, 2020). Once you determine the population and questions, you are ready to get to work in recruiting participants/co-researchers for your photovoice project.

SETTING UP YOUR PROJECT MANAGEMENT PLAN

As described, undertaking any research project, most especially a photovoice project, needs a project management plan. This helps you set up milestones for your research and stay on track throughout in order to be successful. Project management, similar to program management, may be managed through a variety of different forms. There are digital and electronic options such as Jira, Trello, or Excel. Then, there are more traditional methods such as paper-based notes or a whiteboard and colored markers. Choose whatever works for you and your research team. Any plan should include the objectives and activities for your research project, what staff are assigned to those activities, a timeline for completing tasks, and budget information where necessary, and it should be easily accessible to and editable by all team members (Breny, Fagen, & Roe, 2016). At the end, the best-laid plans for your project will come to fruition because you invested time in planning before starting. At the same time, putting a solid system in place prior to implementation allows you to be strategic and flexible enough to make changes when things don't quite go as planned. A sample of a project management plan that was part of a grant proposal requesting funding prior to a photovoice project is provided in the Tools section of this chapter.

RECRUITING PARTICIPANTS

Purposeful sampling of a relatively small group is usually the norm for recruitment for photovoice projects, which aligns with recruitment approaches with most qualitative research. What this means is that that the researcher approaches recruitment with a specific inclusion criterion list of factors, but uses subjectivity and their judgment to select participants that meet the research aims as opposed to recruiting a high number of participants for the goal of yielding generalizable results (Miles et al., 2020; Patton, 2015). This gives you, as the researcher, the ability and flexibility to focus on research aims to include participants whose perspectives lend rich insight into the research topic. It is advisable to recruit a slightly higher number of participants than the ideal for your photovoice project because you can often expect attrition of a few participants. For example, in the past, we aimed to have 15 participants in one study, recruited 21, and retained 16 for the duration of the project. Something else to consider when recruiting for a photovoice project is a reminder that participants are considered your co-researchers. What this means is that you are recruiting with dual roles in mind, which will involve both sharing their own perspectives and opinions and collecting information and doing their best to reflect perspectives of their community or the community of focus for the photovoice study.

As a photovoice project may take place over variable durations ranging from a number of weeks to a number of months, participants must agree to invest ample time, energy, and work into the study. It is usual to request that participants be available for most (if not all) of the photovoice meetings, so appropriately recruiting the right participants is tantamount to your success. It is common to provide incentives to photovoice participants. As we mentioned in Chapter 2, many practitioners and researchers consider incentives such as gift cards a form of remuneration for the work the participants/co-researchers put into the study and we concur with this view.

Depending on the setting for recruitment, posting flyers in spaces with high traffic may be useful. Examples of recruitment flyers used for two of our projects, one with college females and relationship power and the other with Congolese refugee women and their integration and health experiences can be found under Tools at the end of this chapter. When college females reached out to us in response to the flyer, we let them know the expectations right away to help them decide if they wanted to participate. These included that we would have at least five weekly meetings over the course of the semester, they needed to have a smartphone, they needed to be female, and they had to be at least 18 years of age to be selected to participate.

Although reasonably successful, recruiting photovoice participants through "passive" means like a flyer does not always result in the number of people you desire for your project. In many cases, finding a team member to be a recruiter for the project can be invaluable. Ideally, this is someone who is trusted by the community where you are recruiting, someone who works within the community such as a lay health advisor, or someone from a coalition or advisory board who will be better suited to successfully recruit than an unknown researcher (Breny, Lombardi, Madden, & Smoyer, 2017; Delgado, 2015; Rhodes et al., 2015). Given the nature of living in a world with many forms of communication—yet, still feeling disconnected—we have found word-of-mouth recruiting by a known and trusted person to be the most successful. For example, as you will note, the flyer for the recruitment for the study with Congolese refugee women is in English. Having a flyer was desired by the funder, the partner agency, and the particular IRB who approved the study. However, in the end, the primary source of recruitment for that project was a research team member who had a trusting relationship with participants and was able to both literally translate the purpose of the study to their preferred languages and figuratively translate the purpose of the project into relatable terms and concepts.

Many times, you will be working with an existing group (i.e., support group, community coalition, advocacy group) who is ready to take their work further and wants to use photovoice to take some kind of social action. An example of this is one of our photovoice projects that was facilitated through a support group for trans women of color. It started with the leader reaching out to the first author to ask for assistance in conducting a study on the power of gender transitioning (Ruff, Smoyer, & Breny, 2019). This approach can work well as the group is already cohesive and all on board with doing photovoice research. As the researcher, you likely will not have a history with this group and are coming in as the photovoice expert. Your role here will be to earn trust from the group, explain and excite the group on the photovoice method, and guide the photovoice research process. It is still important, however,

FIGURE 3.1

Tips for successful photovoice participant recruitment

Tip 1: Explain exactly what participants will do

Tip 2: Clearly convey how much time is required

Tip 3: Provide incentives for participants

Tip 4: Treat participants as coresearchers and partners throughout the process

---

to get a commitment from group members to attend all the meetings, and, more critical, to give them time to meet for their original purposes, which in this example was the support group. The tips outlined in Figure 3.1 will ensure the successful recruitment and retention of your photovoice participants.

CONSIDERATIONS OF TECHNOLOGY

The nature of photovoice as a visual research method with captured images as its medium necessitates the use of some kind of technology. Comfort with and use of technology will be required throughout your photovoice project—from taking photos during data collection, presenting during analysis, and displaying photos in some way to disseminating results. Next, we guide you through a few considerations of technology.

Cameras and Photography

The choice of what type of cameras to use for photovoice is something to think through carefully. Additionally, photography training is usually included in photovoice project and you will want to determine how lengthy or detailed the training should be based on the needs of the co-researchers. As we have stated, the goal of photovoice is not to produce beautiful, professional photos. Instead, photovoice hinges on the discussions and stories that grow from the photos the participants take. That said, the type of camera you use may be important to the participants if you are providing this as an incentive for their participation, or if one of the goals of your project includes capacity building to provide participants with baseline skills in photography. These are important decisions to make in the planning stages because you only have so much time to do what you need to do to meet your research goals and you want to get it right the first time. Sometimes you may have limited options due to funding restrictions for your project. For example, you may want to buy a certain type of digital camera for all participants, but do not have enough in your budget, or the funder of your photovoice project may have a rule that they do not allow purchases of any type of equipment, which sometimes includes cameras. In such cases, utilizing smartphones that are already in the possession of your participants or using disposable cameras are often the most economical choices. However, if that is not the case, then let us give you some examples of what to consider.

First, consider your audience. Some questions to consider: are they of an age and/or cultural background that they are used to using technology easily? Do they have phones that have a camera? Do they use their camera phones to take pictures regularly? Do they post on social media or upload to websites? Or, are they of an age and place where they might prefer to use cameras without much skill at uploading or posting? Or, are they somewhere in between? Next, consider your project and the social action you hope to achieve (remember, that is the goal of all photovoice projects!). Do you need high-quality photos for websites or for making large prints for public displays, or will the photographs be used solely within the group and displayed using a projector? All of these questions are important to consider.

Using technology that is not appropriate for your audience may lead to unnecessary frustrations in the research process and we have an example from our experience. This particular project involved community lay health advisors exploring social determinants of health related to diabetes and we had a very diverse group of ages with the oldest members in their 70s. All of the participants/co-researchers were women of color living in public housing. The research team, along with the co-researchers, decided to buy everyone a digital single-lens reflex camera. This, it was thought, would be a nice gift to leave with the women as thanks for their participation. The research team hired a professional photographer to train the women to use the cameras over three separate training sessions of two hours each. The sessions were well intended and informative. However, after giving the women a chance to use their cameras to practice we found these sessions overwhelmed them, especially the older participants. In the end, we learned participants preferred a more simple demonstration of the basic steps for how to take the pictures and upload them to send them on to us. Similarly, in the project with Congolese refugee women, some participants had never seen a digital camera, used anything like a camera, and felt intimidated by the process of putting batteries in a camera. Therefore, the training for this project was designed from that as the starting point. The takeaway point here is that you need to know your audience and their comfort levels! Indeed, smartphones have helped facilitate photovoice projects, but just be sure your team of co-researchers have one and know how to use it.

Photo Storage and Displaying

A critical component during later stages of photo discussions and analysis will be to have participant photos easily accessible, which we explain in more detail in Chapter 4. Consider what equipment is available to you and your photovoice project. Will you have access to a computer and projection to show photos during the process? How will you most easily get photos from participants before each meeting? Will they email them to you, bring them on a jump drive, post to a social media site? How will you store them for the duration of your project? Once again, having a well laid out project management plan will help you think through all of the steps in setting up your photovoice project. Additionally, these are potential questions that may also be needed to secure approval through the IRB process we described in Chapter 2. We have used a combination of all of the approaches above such as having participants email the photos to us prior to meetings or uploading the photos on site at the beginning of meetings. For easy retrieval and tracking in the future, we recommend that photos are organized and saved electronically in folders labeled per participant's code name and then, within the folder, the specific photos that participants choose to discuss are also labeled.

CASE ILLUSTRATION—RECRUITMENT, LOGISTICS, AND STARTING A PROJECT

An Interdisciplinary, Photovoice Study With Congolese Refugee Women

To get started, we approached the leadership of a nonprofit agency dedicated to refugee resettlement. It was our hope to initiate a partnership that led to a photovoice project, but the decision was up to the agency. We did a brief presentation about photovoice and then asked whether they felt a photovoice project might be beneficial to them in the work that they do. The agency representatives had several concerns and considerations, particularly in terms of our expectations and ability to work in a respectful, culturally appropriate manner with clients. We had general ideas about subpopulations of refugees of interest as well as general areas of research inquiry, but these were secondary to the needs, interests, and capabilities of the partner agency. After a series of discussions, the partner determined that a photovoice study might enhance the work that they do specifically with women in newer refugee groups to the city in which the study occurred. Together, we applied for external funding from a local agency that prioritized minority health and joint implementation of research between university researchers and community partners. Therefore, the budget allotted the majority of the funding, about 60 percent, to the agency to help offset operational costs and contributed the remainder to the university researchers for implementation of the project.

The mission of the refugee resettlement agency is to support people in the earliest stages of resettlement across all aspects of their lives, so this influenced the development of research questions. Eventually, the resettlement agency and researchers developed general questions centering on understanding the perceptions and experiences of the women in regard to two areas: integration into society U.S. and health care. The latter topic was the interest of the researcher and also was the primary interest of the funder. The partner agency agreed that the results from those questions might help generate information for improving the services of the agency. These research questions were eventually "translated" into two different photo missions. The first, in correspondence with the integration question, was to take photos of things in their lives that make them feel happy, sad, and/or surprised about life in the United States. The second was to take photos of anything in their lives they feel helps or hurts their health, including experiences with health care.

We continued the planning process with a series of discussions between the researchers and the community partner representatives to formulate details together, such as having at least two agency staff members on the research team. We discussed the need for an interpreter and cultural ambassador throughout data collection. Additionally, we planned all aspects of data, such as recruitment of participants, the setting and space where photovoice meetings would be held, and transportation for participants to and from the setting. In this case, the partner agency identified a local community center that was near where most of the study population lived. In terms of transportation, the agency agreed to utilize their van and driver to assist with getting the women to and from photovoice meetings.

We planned all details for five meetings that would last about 3 hours and held over the course of 6 weeks. Plans included approaches to enhance cultural appeal, including Congolese music and food. In this case, we observed that attention to details such as the convenience and comfort of the meeting space, preferred food, and other cultural comforts led to better retention of participants and more open discussion during the phase of photo discussions. Additionally, we made plans to have two laptop computers and a projector available for the meetings when women were returning from their photo mission. This also necessitated building in time for downloading photos and identifying which members of the research team would sit down with participants to upload photos.

The planning stage lasted for about 6 months before we entered the recruitment phase of the project, for which we relied heavily on the partner agency. A flyer was posted at the agency, but since our target population had varying levels of literacy, the research team member who served as the interpreter/cultural ambassador recruited women in person on site at the agency and home-based settings. She identified potential participants, gave them an overview of the study, and then scheduled a time for them to meet with one of the principal investigators for a more detailed description and the informed consent process.

Twenty-one women were recruited for the study over about 2 months and 16 were retained for the duration of the project.

CONCLUSION

There are numerous elements and moving parts to think through when getting started with a photovoice study. As we repeat often in this book, there is going to be great variability in the tasks and steps for getting started depending on the study population, setting, whether you work with a partner or not, research questions, and resources. In this chapter, we covered steps and considerations as you commence your specific photovoice project. Chapter 4 will provide details of implementation, data collection, and ongoing project management.

Chapter 3 Tools

1. Sample Recruitment Flyer: College Women Research

2. Sample Project Management Plan for a Photovoice Study

3. Sample Recruitment Flyer: Photovoice with Congolese Women Research

4. Sample of "Translated" Research Question for Photovoice with Teen Girls

Sample Recruitment Flyer: College Women Research

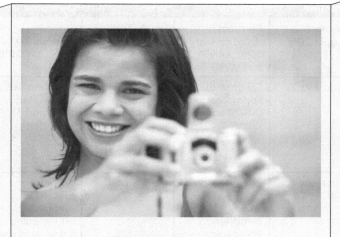

BE A HEALTH RESEARCHER!

ALL YOU NEED IS:

YOUR CAMERA (CELL PHONE CAMERA IS FINE)
YOUR PICTURES
TIME TO MEET FOUR TIMES THIS FALL

And, receive a $25 gift card for your work!
Be a part of a project exploring the nature of relationships, where we get messages of gender roles, and how we can create new messages.
Please be over 18, female, and available this fall.

Sample Project Management Plan for a Photovoice Study

Timeline	Activity	Who	Outcome
July and August 2018	Contract approval with IMHC, UINDY, and WMU	Dr. M, Dr. J, and A.I.	Signed contract by early July 2018
August 2018	Secure IRB approval from UINDY and WMU	Dr. M and university Dr. J and university (All renew CITI certification if expired)	Stamped IRB approval by the start of fall semester in August 2018
September 2018	Identification of the 16 women who actually completed Photovoice in 2016 and recruitment into this study, including scheduling of the interview	Dr. J, Stella	Completion of a study participant list including name, address, phone number, and date and location of where the interview will take place
Early October 2018	Individual interviews including informed consent, survey questions, camera loan, and what we want them to take photos of	Dr. J, Stella	All signed informed consent documents

Timeline	Activity	Who	Outcome
Late October 2018	Collect cameras and download top 3 or 4 photos	Stella and paid research assistant	Cameras are returned and individual electronic folders with all photos from participants are created
November 2018	Conduct 2 focus groups (2 groups of ~8 participants) using the same questions for each and discussing photos	Dr. M, Dr. J, Stella, paid research assistant	Audio files of recorded focus group discussions (1 for each) Written notes from observers of sessions
December 2018– February 2019	Cushion of extra time in case of challenges	All	Finalize study results and submit report to IMHC

Sample Recruitment Flyer: Photovoice with Congolese Women Research

PARTICIPATE IN A PROJECT TO SUPPORT THE HEALTH NEEDS OF YOUR COMMUNITY

(Community partner name) and (university name) are seeking your support in helping us understand social integration and healthcare needs of the Congolese community.

This project will involve taking photographs in your community (camera will be provided). Before taking the photographs, you will be required to participate in an orientation session and a training and practice session. There will be a total of six sessions, each no more than 60 minutes long.

We will provide some refreshments during the session.

Sessions will be held: (insert address). These sessions will take place in March and April 2016 between approximately 6:30 p.m. and 8:00 p.m.

If you are interested, please contact Dr. M (phone/ email) or Dr. J (phone/email).

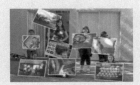

Sample of "Translated" Research Question for Photovoice with Teen Girls

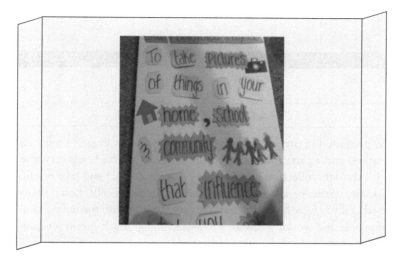

Photovoice Implementation and Data Collection

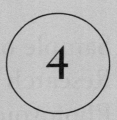

4

CHAPTER OVERVIEW

As presented in previous chapters, photovoice is an iterative research method and a participatory approach to research. This holds very true with the data collection process and it is a process that will take careful planning, patience, and a lot of time. Photovoice data collection is managed as if you were holding a series of focus groups with the same group of people and working toward the project's goal. Each group meeting is important and will have its own agenda and objectives. One goal of the meetings is to foster positive group dynamics as the group proceeds through the photovoice data collection process. Another goal is often to get to the next photo assignment question so that participants can take their pictures and bring them back to discuss. In the end, remember, the goal of photovoice is to give voice to those who haven't been heard and to manage or formulate a plan to take action on the phenomenon under study, so the overarching purpose of the group meeting times is to facilitate and nurture this.

If facilitated effectively, the photovoice data collection process has the potential to simultaneously serve as an educational and empowerment experience or support group. There is potential for participants to build knowledge, skills, social support, and other tools that may be empowering and influence participants to engage as change agents. Conversely, if the data collection process is not well planned or organized in a truly participatory way allowing for substantial flexibility and iteration, then the process has the potential to take voice and power

FIGURE 4.1
Photovoice data collection and analysis process

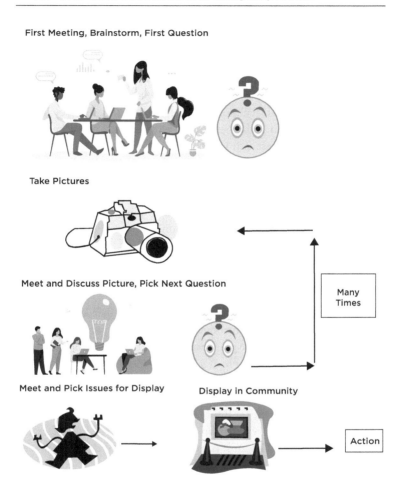

First Meeting, Brainstorm, First Question

Take Pictures

Meet and Discuss Picture, Pick Next Question

Many Times

Meet and Pick Issues for Display

Display in Community

Action

away from participants in the same way that traditional research often does.

In the following section, we describe the steps of the photovoice data collection process as outlined in Figure 4.1, which offers a visual depiction of the iterative process of taking photographs and discussing them in a series of group meetings.

THE CRITICAL FIRST TEAM MEETING

At your first meeting, start from the beginning and be sure to go over the aims of the project and the research questions—if you go the route of already having them. In our experience, every photovoice project is different in how it progresses through the steps of data collection—keep it open and work with your specific group of co-researchers to allow the process to unfold as it will. Participant factors such as age, race, ethnicity, comfort with technology, level of education, literacy levels, language(s) spoken and whether you have interpretation, background, and experience with research will all play a factor in your project and may lead to differences in implementation of photovoice data collection. For some projects, parts of the process may be more prescriptive because of funding or IRB requirements, whereas other projects have more of a blank slate. Your goal, right upfront, is to learn as much as you can about participants while communicating transparently about the participant's roles.

Generally, in this introductory meeting, you will want to dedicate time to building group rapport and supporting everyone to get to know each other. Remember, everyone in the group are co-researchers, so developing a working relationship is important. Other agenda items for this first meeting are to introduce photovoice, discuss logistics, and begin to brainstorm how the group will approach the first photo assignment question. See an example of a First Meeting Agenda in Tools at the end of this chapter.

Indeed, the most important first step at this initial meeting is to create a safe environment for future discussions of pictures and stories, many of which will be very personal and, perhaps, painful. There are many ways to do this. The most common would be to start with an icebreaker that will then lead to establishing group ground rules (Morgan, 2018). One option is to choose an icebreaker activity that is light and fun, for example, have everyone around the room answer a question that has nothing to do with the research topic. Ideas for questions will vary depending on the group, but some possibilities include sharing their favorite food, asking where they would go if they could travel anywhere in the world, or asking what TV show they are streaming/watching at the moment. Another option is to be a bit more serious and ask participants questions designed for self-reflection and learning about each other. For example, the resource offered by the Cultural and Linguistic Community of Practice (2012) offers possibilities such as "cultural introduction" or "cultural scavenger hunt." Selected activities offered in this resource are designed as cultural and linguistic competence icebreakers and may be particularly beneficial if the photovoice participants come from a variety of cultural, racial, ethnic, socioeconomic, or linguistic backgrounds. Go around the table or circle and have everyone answer the question with the ideal of teaching everyone one little thing about each other and increasing the comfort level within the group dynamic. At subsequent meetings, you might ask different questions and use different icebreakers to get the group grounded and ready to start photovoice work.

The next step for the first meeting is to establish group ground rules. Setting ground rules for any group is crucial—and even more so for a photovoice project, as participants will be working closely with each other on sensitive topics for several weeks. Usually and ideally, ground rules are established by the group. You start with a blank piece of newsprint or whiteboard and ask the group to suggest ground rules that everyone will adhere to for the duration of the photovoice project. However, you can also feel free to begin the list and have the group brainstorm more. To begin, you may want to establish ground rules around privacy and confidentiality of others' stories and experiences; respect of one another; a commitment to staying involved with the project moving forward; and the freedom to ask any question without fear. Having the group "own" these rules is integral to the photovoice project's success.

Once the stage is set, and ground rules established, the first meeting is integral for explaining the purpose of the research project. Be clear and honest about the goals of your research, present contextual data if that will help your participants see your mission, and find out any information they may have about the research project goals. For example, when working with a group of college students embarking on a project to increase condom use, we found it was important to present data to the group on sexually transmitted infection (STI) rates among college students nationally and condom use rates from campus-based surveys to help set the stage for initiating the project (Breny & Lombardi, 2017). At the same time, remember to urge participants to stay focused.

Make sure to emphasize that this is, indeed, research, and their pictures and words will be the data to be analyzed. Clarify that any questions they may have will be answered.

Depending on your audience, discussions about photography and photojournalism may be important to explain. Be aware not to spend too much time on the details of taking a good photograph as that might take participant's focus away from the photo assignment question they will be using for your next meeting. At this initial meeting, it is important to introduce the important point that the quality of photos is not as important as the discussions people will have about those photos and to reinforce this message in subsequent meetings. The main message to communicate is, "There are no wrong pictures!"

For some groups, you may need to introduce them to using cameras and taking photos. For other groups, you might just review the basics of taking photos, encouraging them to find things to photograph that have meaning for them. This overview of camera use may be included in the first meeting or may need to be scheduled into a future meeting, depending mainly on how much time you have for the project. Discuss issues around release forms for photos of people, and encourage them to take pictures that do not show people's faces to reduce challenges with some of the aforementioned privacy concerns. Once you have reviewed the goals of the research project and created a safe environment for group discussions, you can now turn to facilitate a discussion that will result in your first photo assignment for the next meeting. This is done by having the group brainstorm ideas and issues that might pertain to the project's research aims.

As a group leader, you will facilitate that discussion in the direction of posing a question for photo exploration, one that is broad enough to allow for multiple perspectives but simple enough so that participants can take photos that illustrate their responses to it. For example, the first question for a project with men about condom-use responsibility could be: "What are the roles of men and women in relationships?" This question is both broad and specific and is a starting-off point for more specific questions on safer-sex communication and negotiation. When the question is agreed to by all, schedule the next meeting in a week or two, and ask participants to bring in a set number of photos to share with the group. It is important to communicate at least an estimated number of photos that you are expecting and to communicate the importance of the deadline for taking the photos because these are areas that may lead to delays in the project timeline if there is confusion or miscommunication. For example, during one of our projects, we did not specify how many photos we recommended the participants take and they returned their cameras with an average of just five photos. This led to extending the timeline for the project because the participants were then encouraged to take an additional week to take at least 10 photos. A good rule to follow, to help keep the project moving forward, is to ask participants to bring two to three photos to share with the group each time you meet. A sample agenda for a first photovoice meeting can be found in Tools at the end of this chapter.

Again, it must be emphasized that the group members or the topic of your photovoice project may lead to variation in the approach to your first meeting. For example, in one project with undergraduate college male students (Breny & Lombardi, 2017), the first meeting of the photovoice research team actually involved discussion around whether or not the participants (male) would be comfortable discussing topics around safer sex and gender norms with the researchers (female). We discussed it at length, the researchers left the room to let the participants make their decisions, and their conclusion was that they were just fine with female researchers facilitating the discussions. The lesson of this is that photovoice is very personal and it is important that your participants feel completely comfortable discussing their pictures and the meanings of these pictures in the group discussions. To set the stage for doing just that at your first meeting is critical.

OPTION FOR PREPARATION MEETINGS PRIOR TO PHOTO QUESTIONS

Depending on the population you are working with, time, and resources available, it may be advantageous to have a series of preparation meetings. For example, when working with vulnerable, marginalized groups, we have found that engaging in multiple meetings prior to participants heading out for their "photo mission" is helpful for building both rapport and a solid foundation for your photovoice research. Below is a sample schedule of photovoice meetings that was followed with Congolese refugee women in a community setting. Another, more extensive sample of meetings and topics for a project with teen girls is included in the Tools at the end of the chapter. Note that the number of sessions and times are certainly different, which illustrates how photovoice projects vary and are tailored to the group, time, setting, and resources that you have.

1. Prep Meeting 1: Ground rules/rapport building: about 2 hr

2. Prep Meeting 2: Cameras 101: Camera distribution, hands-on training, and practice around the community center: about 3 hr

3. Prep Meeting 3: Ethics, safety, and security: about 2 hr

4. Prep Meeting 4: Final preparation, reviewing the photo mission, and confirming the next steps: about 1 hr

For some projects, it may be beneficial to provide food and facilitate the meetings in a comfortable, welcoming space to help participants feel safe. For example, the aforementioned photovoice project with Congolese refugee women was held in a community center near the homes of most of the participants (McMorrow & Saksena, 2017; Saksena & McMorrow, 2019). Flexibility and the expectation for variation are key elements required when facilitating a series of photovoice meetings. Again, the ideal is to collaborate with participants as co-researchers at every stage of the process, so engaging them in decision making about the logistics of photovoice meetings (time, frequency, space, food, format) enhances rapport building and ultimately retention of participants for the duration of the project. For this particular project, culturally appealing food and music were included throughout all of the meetings.

Meetings to Discuss Photos

The subsequent meetings to discuss photos and choose a follow-up question should be simpler and more straightforward than the first orientation and brainstorming meeting. These meetings are intended to contextualize and understand the meanings of the photographs taken by participants (Wang & Burris, 1997). In essence, your role will be to facilitate dialogue among the group, listen to what they are saying about their photographs, and help to contextualize their meaning. The ideal is for discussions of photos to be audio- or video-recorded with participant consent and transcribed later, which serves as a major portion of your data. It is recommended that the photo discussion meetings are, at a minimum, audio-taped and transcribed (Breny, Lombardi, Madden, & Smoyer, 2017).

Based on Freirean methods of achieving critical consciousness and tenets of feminist theory, as we have previously mentioned, photovoice is a process that allows participants to dialogue about the root causes of the phenomenon under study (Wang & Burris, 1994, 1997; Wang, Burris, & Ping, 1996). The way in which you achieve that in your group is up to you; however, there are methods by which you can do this, such as, the SHOWeD technique of questioning (Breny et al., 2017; Seitz & Strack, 2016; Wang, Morrel-Samuels, Hutchinson, Bell, & Pestrock, 2004). For each picture the participant has chosen to present, you as facilitator may ask the following series of questions:

1. What do you *S*ee here?

2. What is really *H*appening?

3. How does this relate to *O*ur lives?

4. *W*hy does this problem or strength exist?

5. What can we *D*o about it?

You can see that this series of questions does two things. First, it gets to the core meanings of the photo being presented (and any issues or assets associated with that), and it facilitates the discussion toward how to use this photo and its meaning to make change. There are other series of questions you can, of course, use while your participants discuss your photos but it will be most helpful to use the same series of questions for each photograph for analysis purposes. Another option for questioning is the acronym PHOTO (Hussey, 2006):

1. Describe your *P*icture

2. What is *H*appening in your picture?

3. Why did you take a picture *Of* this?

4. What does this picture *T*ell us about your life?

5. How can this picture make a p*O*sitive change?

Use whatever process will work best for you.

For this and subsequent photo discussion meetings, you will facilitate the questioning process for each participant and their group of photos. You may want to discuss anywhere from the top two photos selected by each participant to 10 photos, depending on the size of the group. However, it is recommended that you do not attempt to discuss more than 10 photos or you may run out of time to discuss them.

During discussions about participant photos, anyone in the group can ask follow-up questions to further delve into and explore root issues/strengths of the photos. If possible, it may be useful during data collection to facilitate the photo discussions similar to how one would facilitate a focus group in that you encourage participants to talk with each other and build off of what others are saying. For example, Participant A may answer the SHOWeD questions and then you might ask whether others had a similar photo and if so, prompt them to share more about the similarities and differences in their responses to SHOWeD. Or, another question could be whether anyone had taken a photo that reflected a similar issue. Sometimes participants may interject and speak up to say that they had the same photo or that they have had a similar experience as another participant. Go with this! Sometimes you may feel like you need to stick to the research script, but that is the beauty of an iterative, flexible method like photovoice. It can be powerful when participants realize they are not the only one with a specific experience or perspective. This may then lead to the group learning, support, and empowerment that is possible with photovoice. Facilitation of the photovoice discussions to nurture and inspire dialogue beyond the surface of the photos will enhance data collection. After everyone has spoken about his/her photos, a final step might be to brainstorm or discuss parameters for the next photograph assignment, if there is another one, as was done in the initial meeting.

An additional tool that may enhance your data collection process is to have participants journal their photo meanings and personal process during the weeks they are taking pictures (Madden & Breny, 2016). This might be done in a traditional, written format. Or, taking literacy levels, language preference, and the participant's comfort level with writing, another way to approach "journaling" could be to have participants orally share their reflections and process and record them on their smartphone if they have one. If the primary language of the project is English and participants choose another language for recording their "journals," then translation may be necessary. As there may be a span of a week or two between photovoice meetings, you will want to be sure to capture all of their thoughts and perceptions and a journal process might be ideal for this. Recommend participants record their thoughts about each photo during the week and then share whatever they want to at the meetings. These journals, either written or recorded, can be analyzed further during data analysis. However, this is something you want to decide about before commencing your photovoice study and think through the process thoroughly in order to include it in your IRB application.

Potential Challenges to Implementation

The process of implementation that has been described is, of course, an ideal. In terms of the suggested meetings, there is a possibility and perhaps even likelihood that they will not go as planned, much in the same way that teachers encounter challenges in the classroom or a youth development worker has to pivot when facilitating groups in community settings. Conflict may occur between participants or between you and the participants. Therefore, it is important to consider this possibility and have a plan in case conflict occurs. Ideally, you or the team members leading photovoice meetings have a baseline of skill in group facilitation. If not, it may be beneficial to read or undergo brief training in the basics (Community Toolbox, Chap. 16; Morgan, 2018). In our experience, the aforementioned recommendations for building rapport and setting group norms at the outset of the project have helped greatly with minimizing conflict, but we both have a background of group facilitation and teaching that likely enabled us to manage conflict with relative ease.

In addition to expecting conflict, there is also the chance that scheduled photovoice meetings do not go as planned because of illness, weather, unexpected logistical challenges, or simply because participants are human and may end up having different priorities or goals for the photovoice meetings in spite of your best planning efforts. For example, we once planned an initial meeting to follow up with a population for a second photovoice study after they had completed one 3 years earlier. We built in 3 hours for the meeting. However, that fell short of the time we required to both truly reconnect with the participants to reignite trust and to collect data in a focus group setting. In that scenario, we ended at the time we stated we would end, primarily because the participants held us accountable in saying they had to leave because their transportation had arrived. There was less data than we expected to collect from that session, but in the end, there was still enough data and we had prioritized trust building that set the scene for a more successful second meeting.

Despite photovoice being considered a community-based participatory research method that views participants as co-researchers, there is still an implicit power differential that is important to acknowledge. It may lead participants to feel inclined to defer to you as the researcher. Therefore, a common challenge present in the photovoice data collection process is that participants might take photos of things they think *you* want them to photograph rather than things they truly feel compelled to capture. This is a form of participant bias, sometimes described as social desirability bias (Nyamathi & Shuler, 1990) that is common in research. In a photovoice project, this is of particular concern because it is counter to the stated goal of using photovoice as a forum for participants who may not often be given space to share their perspectives and experiences that are underrepresented. If they end up censoring the photos they take and/or discuss because they believe the researcher does not want to see them or hear about them, then it may contribute to a cycle of suppressing voices of the population. This may be a threat to the credibility of your research (Tolley, Ulin, Mack, Robinson, & Succup, 2016) because both photos and subsequent discussions may end up diluting the question(s) you and the co-researchers have set out to answer. We have found this to be a challenge when facilitating photovoice across a range of populations.

One way to reduce this form of bias is constant, repetitive reassurance for participants that the primary purpose of the research is seeing and hearing *their* point of view through taking and subsequently discussing photos of anything and everything that they feel fits within the photo assignment. As mentioned earlier, there are absolutely no "wrong" photos and it is important to communicate this early and often with participants. Another way to attempt to minimize social desirability bias is to be frank and honest during the initial stages of forming group norms about recognition of your positionality, inherent privileges, and differentials of power (Nyamathi & Shuler, 1990; Patton, 2015; Tolley et al., 2016) as the researcher. Additionally, it may be beneficial to be forthright in naming other characteristics that may compound these socially constructed power differentials such as adults working with youth, a white person working with people of color, or a researcher born in the United States working with people who are immigrants.

Another challenge that may occur during data collection is when participants return photos, you find a significantly different number of photos than expected. Depending on the population you are working with, it may help to give participants a rough guideline for how many photos to take. For example, if you are using disposable cameras, then perhaps you might recommend that they take all 24 or 36 photos. Sometimes, despite successful preparation meetings and giving a guideline for the number of photos, participants might return from the photo assignment with the feedback that it just did not work for them or; that they did not encounter things in their environment that aligned with the photo assignment during the time period for photo taking. This can be a significant challenge if you have a tight timeline or budget, but it is something to recognize as a possibility.

In terms of communicating with people who may end up being "subjects" of photos, one possibility is to prepare laminated cards in advance that spell out the reason for the photovoice project and include your information as the researcher. If participants encounter a challenging situation with someone asking a lot of questions about why they are taking photos, they can simply share the card and encourage the person to contact the lead researcher. This method was used with Congolese refugee women who had limited English skills and although it seemed they did not need to use the cards during data collection, it was helpful in reassuring participants that the cards were there to fall back on in case they felt uncomfortable or threatened (McMorrow & Saksena, 2017; Saksena & McMorrow, 2019).

CASE STUDY TO ILLUSTRATE IMPLEMENTATION

Although photovoice data collection generally follows the guidelines and processes we have been discussing, it is important to recognize that there can and often will be diversity between projects. Also, things likely will not go as planned. It is certainly true that the photovoice data collection process of one researcher will vary from another researcher, but additionally, the authors have found there to be notable differences each time they lead or contribute to photovoice study. Again, factors such as time, resources, population you are working with, area of research inquiry, funding sources, or even unexpected events in the greater sociopolitical landscape may lead to unique steps or iterations in your process. Here we offer one example of a scenario of the photo data collection process from our research to illustrate potential steps you may take with your process and also to show the range of possibilities that may occur during the process.

In much of the research literature as in society, negative connotations come to people's minds with regard to transgender individuals that are based on fear, ignorance, and/or lack of experience with this population. Although the media coverage of Caitlin Jenner several years ago raised awareness of the positive truths and realities of living as a transgender individual, legislation restricting bathroom access, for example, increased negative stereotypes and poor treatment of people who are transgender. Indeed, disproportionately high rates of HIV, sexually transmitted diseases, alcohol use, and substance are seen among transgender men and women (Baral et al., 2013; Hughes & Eliason, 2002; Sausa, Keatley, & Operario, 2007; Sevelius, Keatley, & Gutierrez-Mock, 2011). Further, high rates of mental health issues, depression, and suicidal tendencies affect this population strongly because of the way society views and mistreats them (Clements-Nolle, Marx, & Katz, 2006). Members of the transgender community are also at higher risk of being victims of violence, sometimes because of their experiences working as sex workers in high crime neighborhoods (Operario, Soma, & Underhill, 2008). The injustice of disproportionate violence and murder of transgender women of color continues in society today.

Not surprisingly, support groups for people who are transgender are common. This particular project was initiated within an existing support group of transgender women of color that was led by a social work student (a trans woman of color) from the local community (Ruff, Smoyer & Breny, 2019). The support group met regularly to provide moral support and referrals to women who had already transitioned or were in the process of doing so. The leader of the support group learned about the photovoice method in a social work research methods course she took and presented it to the group as a method to use to share their experiences of transitioning with an emphasis on adding positive realities of living as transgender to the literature. She employed a social work professor and one of the authors to be co-principal investigators on the project. Here we describe how data collection was conducted in this project.

At the first meeting to discuss photovoice, the women were given an article to read on the purpose and process of conducting a photovoice project. A full discussion about how to take photos, how many photos to take, release forms for any people in the pictures, and other details were facilitated by the group leader and the two faculty members present. The group concluded with a clear understanding of the research process and the assignment to bring in a picture illustrating their experiences transitioning to becoming a woman.

Five women agreed to participate in the photovoice project: three were Black and two were Latinx. Weekly, 2-hour meetings were convened, for 7 weeks, to share and discuss photos. Because participants were from an already existing support group, the conversation flowed easily and women were comfortable sharing experiences. Women expressed how they had been treated in society. Much of the discussion in the meetings centered on supporting each other through their trials and tribulations, being denied work, being laughed out of city hall when trying to change their gender on their driver's license, and getting labeled as the wrong sex when admitted to the hospital. These conversations became the fodder for the photos that would eventually be brought into the group meetings.

The process was designed intentionally so that each week a different woman would bring in her pictures to share and discuss. Interestingly, each woman brought just one or two very thoughtful pictures with them to the group meeting, mainly because of the rich discussions they already had in previous meetings. For this project, photos were brought on cell phones and shared with the group as they told their stories of why the pictures were taken. Despite some conversations around

FIGURE 4.2

Of this picture, the co-researcher said,

"This is where I want to be in the next 5 years. I want to be married with the picket fence and everything like, so that's what that means basically. I feel like I'm already 75 percent there, I just gotta find the husband and the house. Or I might not even find the husband, I just want the house....I just want to live a normal life as a citizen." She continues to talk about the desire to have a "normal life."

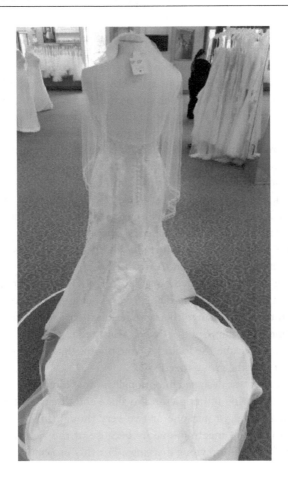

negative treatments and frustrations of transitioning, the photos were of strengths, namely resilience, hope, and courage brought to fruition by the support they had received from their "sisters" in previous meetings Ruff, Smoyer, & Breny, 2019). For each picture, the photovoice SHOWeD technique was conducted by the group leader (Wang & Burris, 1997).

An example of a photo taken and the explanation of the photo in Figure 4.2 is an image of a wedding dress taken by a woman who was engaged, and then the engagement broken off by the man to whom she was engaged.

The final meeting consisted of "member checking" or the process of sharing and confirming results with participants in order to get validation for accuracy (Guba, 1981). The way this often works in photovoice is sharing the photos and accompanying stories such as the previous example and asking participants if this accurately captures what they shared or meant to communicate. This meeting was held in a different location from the rest, in a beautiful office space 10 floors about the town green, with a beautiful view of the city. Catered food was offered at the meeting to set the stage for a celebratory finish to the photovoice project. It was powerful and moving to watch the women as they saw their photos and words come to life in a PowerPoint presentation. Many were moved to tears and several added even more context to their pictures this second time around. It was clear that the sheer process of being a participant in this research project, and the power of photovoice, gave these women strength as a community to fully stand in their power as transgender women.

CONCLUSION

It cannot be overemphasized that the photovoice data collection process has the *potential* to positively impact participants and engage as change agents but only if the implementation process is thoughtfully and intentionally carried out with this goal in mind. As noted, ongoing flexibility and iteration are keys to success. Building in elements of all photovoice group meetings to cultivate rapport and support participant empowerment will ease implementation and enhance the experience for all involved. As we move on to Chapter 5, we will concentrate on presenting options and introductory steps for analyzing and displaying photovoice data.

Chapter 4 Tools

1. Sample of a First Meeting Agenda

2. Sample of Agendas, Topics, and Curriculum for All Sessions

Sample of a First Meeting Agenda

A generic agenda for this first meeting could be:

1. Introductions/icebreaker

2. Establishing group ground rules

3. Overview of research aims/questions

4. Logistics

   a. How to take photos/number of photos to take

   b. Frequency and overview of upcoming meetings

   c. How meetings will be facilitated

   d. Communication among team members

5. Brainstorming first photo assignment

6. Wrap-up/reminder of next meeting

Sample of Agendas, Topics, and Curriculum for All Sessions

PRE-SESSION: PARENT/GUARDIAN AND YOUTH PARTICIPANTS ATTEND INFORMATIONAL AND CONSENT SESSION

Estimated time: 30 minutes to 1 hour
    Setting: Saginaw High School–Based Health Center
    Time: After-school hours or evening
    Goals:

- Explain photovoice

- Explain roles and time commitment for participants

- Explain who is involved (funders and sponsoring organizations)

- Give estimated timeline of the project

- Review of fact sheet and consent forms

- Question and answer

- Meet the project staff

- Go over consent forms

- Participants and parents/guardians turn in consent and assent forms

Session 1: Introductory Meeting With Youth Participants

Estimated time: 45 minutes
    Setting: Saginaw High School Media Center

Time: Lunch period during school hours
Goals:

- Introductions
- Create project ground rules
- Understanding photovoice/the project—Intro
- Plan for the rest of the project

Session 2: Photovoice Training

Estimated time: 45 minutes
  Setting: Saginaw High School Media Center
  Time: Lunch period during school hours
  Goals:

- Understanding photovoice/the project—continued
- Photography Power, Ethics, and Legal Issues
  - ○ Overview of image ethics: intrusion into private space, disclosure of embarrassing facts about individuals, being placed in false light by images, protection against the use for commercial benefit
  - ○ Explain consent forms for people who may be photographed
  - ○ Explain the ethics of photo-taking form

Session 3: Photovoice Training

Estimated time: 45 minutes
  Setting: Saginaw High School Media Center
  Time: Lunch period during school hours
  Goals:

- Cameras 101
- Photography 101

○ Guest speaker: local photographer

Session 4: Community Photo Practice Session

Estimated time: 45 minutes
    Setting: To be determined; near Saginaw High School campus
    Time: Lunch period during school hours
    Goals:

- Practice using the cameras

- Remind participants of photovoice ethics

Session 5: Debriefing of Practice Session and Assignment for Official Upcoming Photovoice Session

Estimated time: 45 minutes
    Setting: Saginaw High School Media Center
    Time: Lunch period during school hours
    Goals

- Discuss lessons learned from practice session

- Review of photovoice ethics

- Directions for the next round of official photo taking: distribution of cameras, labeling of cameras, participants take a photo of themselves, participants review ethics of photovoice form, participants agree to bring the cameras back for the next meeting in 2 weeks

- Distribute consent forms for people who may be photographed

- Answer questions

Session 6: Reflection Meeting #1

Estimated time: 45 minutes
    Setting: Saginaw High School Media Center

Time: Lunch period during school hours
Goals:

- Participants will be divided into two groups of four; each will have an SVSU facilitator
- Participants will remove any personal photos, go over the photovoice photos, fill out the photo consent form to identify which photos can be used by SVSU/HDI
- Choose 10 most significant photos
- Start individual reflection on SHOWeD questions

Session 7: Reflection Meeting #2: SHOWED Questions in Focus Groups

Estimated time: 1 to 2 hours
Setting: Saginaw High School Media Center
Time: To be determined
Goals:

- Participants will return to the same groups as Reflection meeting #1
- Review ground rules
- Participants will narrow down their top 10 photos to 3 favorite/most significant photos
- Each SVSU facilitator will take the participants through focus group discussions of the photos using the SHOWeD questions

Session 8: Reflection Meeting #3: Storytelling Session

Estimate time: 1 to 2 hours
Setting: Saginaw High School Media Center
Time: To be determined
Goals:

- Participants process their top three photos in the large group by sharing and identifying themes

- Participants select two photos and document their stories with captions

- Participants are led through a facilitated discussion on ways to take action on the issues and themes in their photos

Session 9: Preparation for Celebration/Public Display

Estimated time: 45 minutes
  Setting: Saginaw High School Media Center
  Time: Lunch period during school hours

- Confirm celebration/public display date, time, location

- Assign distribution of fliers, emails, phone calls to invite policymakers and decisions in the community

- Organize all other arrangements for celebration/public display

CELEBRATION/PUBLIC DISPLAY

Session 10: Closing Debriefing Session and Final Interviews

Estimated time: 2 hours
  Setting: Saginaw High School Media Center and SHSHC exam
room
  Time: To be determined

- Closing remarks and gratitude from project staff and participants

- Individual interviews of each of the eight participants conducted by each of the SVSU facilitators

Analyzing and Presenting Photovoice Data

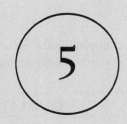

The core requisites for qualitative analysis (are) a little creativity, systematic doggedness, some good conceptual sensibilities and cognitive flexibility.
—HUBERMAN AND MILES (1994, P. 17)

CHAPTER OVERVIEW

In this chapter, we introduce the basics of photovoice data analysis and options for sharing photovoice results to create the biggest impact on social change. Our aims are twofold. First, we walk you through the academic approach for analyzing and presenting data, particularly in the context of traditional venues for dissemination such as conferences and manuscripts. Additionally, we offer ideas for following through on the component of action to reach policymakers that were critical to the original conception of photovoice by Wang, Burris, and Ping (1996) and Wang and Burris (1997). Arguably, action for advocacy is the most crucial step for utilizing photovoice for social justice, but presenting photovoice data with intentional, concerted action for social change seems to have been somewhat diluted by various researchers using photovoice over time. This is likely because of a myriad of reasons such as limited resources, lack of knowledge or skill for implementing action, and the misplaced value of academic presentation versus community change. However, in keeping with the focus of this book on photovoice as a means to advocate for social justice, this chapter culminates with examples illustrating how photovoice data were used both for presentation in academic settings and for advocating for social change.

QUALITATIVE DATA ANALYSIS

First and foremost, it is important to describe qualitative data analysis and how it differs from quantitative data analysis. Briefly, quantitative data analysis is *deductive* in nature and requires that researchers choose their variables and expected outcomes a priori, or in advance. Conversely, qualitative research is usually conducted *inductively*, meaning that researchers go into their studies with the intention of exploring their data for emerging themes that explain a given phenomenon under investigation through their research questions (Tolley, Ulin, Mack, Robinson, & Succop, 2016). Once your first focus group, interview, or photovoice session is conducted, the reviewing of transcripts and data commences as you search for themes and directions for the next round of data collection. In this way, qualitative analysis is iterative, allowing for researchers to build upon what they are learning for upcoming data collection, always keeping in mind the original research aim and intent of the project as you move forward (Huberman & Miles, 1994).

Figure 5.1 is just one of many ways to visualize the iterative process of analyzing qualitative data (Tolley et al., 2016). We present this to you as a primer for understanding the photovoice data analysis process. You see that the first two steps, "reading" and "coding," are done while you are still in the data collection process, emphasizing again that you begin analysis from the very start of data collection. The "reading" step requires that you read (or listen to) transcripts and review photos for both content and relevance to your research aims and also for themes or patterns in the discussions that could later become "codes." Step 2 is "coding" your data, which is done while you are reading and getting familiar with it. Codes are "like street signs inserted into the margins of" your transcripts or notes from the photovoice meetings (Tolley et al., 2016, p. 179). These codes will be organized later to give you your overall results, but in the short term, they are ways for you to clearly note common themes in the data. You can set up codes according to your research questions or as they emerge from the data organically.

Steps 3 and 4, "displaying" and "reducing," are conducted once you have read and coded all of your transcripts and photos. These steps

FIGURE 5.1

Example of the Qualitative Data Analysis Process

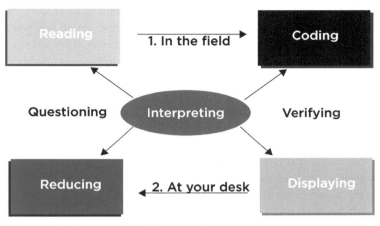

Source: Tolley et al. (2016, p. 176).

will give you the ability to see the actual findings of your research project. Displaying the data means that you lay out your coded data, so you can now begin to seek out subthemes within the codes. You are crafting a hypothesis or theory of how you will answer the research questions and take the next step to action. Once there, you will reduce the data to see the relationships between all of these codes to fully understand the big picture in your project (Tolley et al., 2016). We provide more detail on this in the following pages.

PARTICIPATORY ANALYSIS

Participants are viewed as co-researchers with photovoice projects. What does that mean and how does it really work? From a research project implementation perspective, there is great variation throughout all stages of photovoice. For some photovoice projects, researchers may take the lead on data analysis while encouraging participants to take the lead in other stages of planning the study, refining the research question, and taking photos as well as the latter stages of planning for a public display of the photos. Another approach is for the lead researcher to facilitate participant co-researchers through a process of training and learning skills in data analysis. As with all stages of a photovoice project, it is important to keep the lines of communication open for participants and researchers to work together to determine comfort levels of involvement in data analysis of participants. For example, an academic researcher conducting photovoice as part of their research toward tenure or promotion may have a more complex and time-consuming data analysis plan for which participant co-researchers do not want to commit time. On the other hand, a different academic researcher, a social worker, a community health educator, or a community development professional may be using photovoice as a means to build capacity and critical consciousness of participants. In the latter examples, participants may contribute to all portions of data analysis to enhance their knowledge and skills and to add a valuable layer of insight and richness to the photovoice analysis.

It has been noted that the photovoice literature is sparse in terms of publications spelling out how to conduct analysis of photovoice data (Capous-Desyllas & Broomfield, 2018). Other literature describing photovoice allude to the fact that participants contributed to analysis but is vague about *how* they participated (Fortin, Jackson, Maher, & Moravac, 2015), so it is important to be clear and explicit about the role of participants in the analysis process. One approach we have used is to have participants be solely responsible for choosing which photographs they want to discuss with fellow participants in recorded discussions. After participants take photos, the next step can be for participants to choose their top photos to share and describe with the group. The number allotted for top choices will vary depending on the size of the group and the length of time available for discussions of photos. One possibility is to ask participants to choose two or three of their top photos while remaining open and flexible if they only want to discuss one, or they end up having four or five they feel strongly about sharing. This is a more participatory approach and often leads to longer photo discussion sessions. For example, when we had 10 women in one study who discussed two or three photos, the session took about 3 hours. Sometimes researchers do not have the luxury of time, so in that case, there may be a need for a more traditional approach with the researcher as the primary decision maker requesting participants choose only one or two photos and discussing a maximum of two in a given session.

Another more traditional and less participatory approach may view having the participants choosing the photos as a potential loss or waste of data in terms of the photos that the participant does not choose. Researchers might examine all of the photos and make the decisions about which photos will be discussed. However, in our view, this approach to analysis is not well aligned with the ethos of photovoice and excludes participants from the analysis process. Other times, researchers may guide participants through discussion of photos they select but then go on to analyze photos that participants did not choose for discussion. This option is more participatory than the former. However, the underlying idea of photovoice is that photos alone do not yield rich information without the power of the participant's choice to share that photo and the accompanying narrative data.

PHOTOVOICE ANALYSIS PROCESS

As we discussed in Chapter 3, discussions of selected photos employing the SHOWeD or similar method should be audio-recorded at a minimum, with participant consent. Video recording is another excellent option to provide additional data of nonverbal facial expressions, body language, and interactions between the participants and the researchers. Either way, the result is often several hours of recording that then needs to be transcribed verbatim. Some researchers choose to transcribe recordings as part of the process of immersing themselves in the data, whereas others employ a transcription service. Either way, transcription of photovoice discussions often results in many pages of transcribed data that could be anywhere from 20 to over 100 pages long. The next step may be to apply qualitative data analysis techniques to organize and make sense of the interview transcripts in conjunction with the photos. Examples of possible qualitative analysis techniques that have been used successfully with photovoice data are qualitative content analysis (McMorrow & Saksena, 2017), constant comparison analysis (Strack, Aronson, Orsini, Seitz, & McCoy, 2018), grounded theory (López, Eng, Randall-David, & Robinson, 2005), visual ethnography (Carlson, Engebretson, & Champberlain, 2006), and thematic analysis (Braun & Clarke, 2006; Breny & Lombardi, 2017).

Something that differentiates analysis of photovoice discussion transcripts from general analysis of focus group discussions is that the researcher must always keep in mind the photo or photos that sparked the discussion. Analysis of visual data as the primary focus in a research project is deserving of a stand-alone book. Miles, Huberman, and Saldana offer a helpful introduction and several resources to become acquainted with approaches to visual data analysis (2020). However, for the purposes of photovoice and limitations of this book, we consider the visual data as inextricably tied to the narrative data, and in some ways, the visual data might be considered secondary. For the analysis process, the photos should be labeled and accessible for an iterative review in conjunction with analyzing the photovoice discussion transcripts. Simultaneously, the notes and coding of the data in the transcripts often extend to the photos as well.

Some photovoice researchers choose to conduct separate analyses of photos and transcripts followed by triangulation of these as two data sources (Carlson et al., 2006). Other researchers analyze the photovoice transcripts with the goal of forming the data into a caption or story to accompany each photo in the data set that was selected by participants. This is an approach we have taken that has worked well. In this scenario, a critical component of at least one of the photovoice group meetings toward the end of the project after analysis has occurred is to engage in member checking (Creswell, 2015; Denzin & Guba, 2017). This involves presenting the selected photos along with the accompanying story or caption that has emerged from analysis to the participants for the purpose of making sure the data accurately represents what the participants were voicing both with taking the photo and the story. Additionally, it is recommended to work with participants to modify the stories as required and engage in ongoing informed consent to ensure that participants are still comfortable with sharing the selected photos and stories.

Again, qualitative data analysis is done by reviewing the data for common themes or storylines that can be categorized to show a summary of the truths being presented by the research. Many qualitative researchers find using qualitative analysis software or web-based programs a convenient way to organize their data. However, it is important to recognize that these are data management tools with limitations; you, the participants/co-researchers, and other research team members are the true analyzers. For those interested in learning about management software, there are several popular choices ranging in cost and

FIGURE 5.2

Example from Photovoice Study with Congolese Women

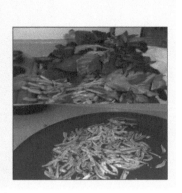

DAILY EXPERIENCES OF
HEALTH

"That this is a vegetable, one of the
vegetables from Africa, it is called dodo. They
have obligated me at the doctor to eat a lot
of vegetables from home that I know, but it
is very, very hard to find in this country. He
didn't say this specific one, but he told me
vegetables, and this is what I know
vegetables is…they have been
imported…but it is so hard to find"

"It is a dry fish, it is a very good nutrition
that I know, but the purpose of taking the
picture, it is so rare we cannot find it here.
It is a dry fisth, but it is very nutritious and
very good for you. It is always expensive or
hard to find it"

ease of use, which are NVivo (Nvivo, 2018), Atlas.ti, Dedoose, and HyperResearch (HyperResearch, 2013), to name a few.

Taking the general process of qualitative analysis a few steps farther, we describe this brief, three-step process of inductive coding, which means starting with the raw data. The steps are organizing and initial analysis, establishment of codes, and establishment of themes. Figures 5.2–5.5 are examples of the final goal you are working toward with photovoice analysis, so we offer these as images for you to consider as you read through the following steps.

Organizing and Initial Analysis

- Read thoroughly through the full transcript for a first time after you've read transcripts for each group meeting along the way.

- Highlight the content in the transcript, clearly noting which participants shared each different story and narrative section. One simple way to clarify which participant shared which story is color coding throughout the transcript by having one color for each of the participants.

FIGURE 5.3
Photovoice for Commmunity Action

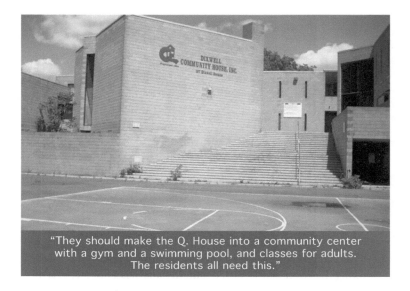

"They should make the Q. House into a community center with a gym and a swimming pool, and classes for adults. The residents all need this."

- Code and organize the photos that were discussed so that you are able to readily reference them in correspondence with each of the distinct stories from each participant. For example, imagine you highlighted the three stories of Participant A in yellow where she described one photo of a car, one photo of a television, and one photo of a bag of groceries. You will want to label each photo accordingly, so you might also use yellow and label them in a way that you can easily refer back to them when you read the data again such as "Participant A Car," "Participant A TV," "Participant A Groceries," or a simple number system such as "Participant A Photo 1," etc.

- Return to the transcript again to update the highlighted sections by adding the photo labels you have chosen. Again, your goal is to establish an easy process for iteratively going back and forth between reading the narrative data and viewing the visual data during the next round of analysis.

FIGURE 5.4

Example from Photovoice Study with Congolese Women

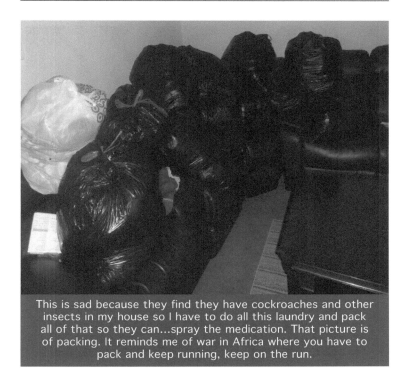

This is sad because they find they have cockroaches and other insects in my house so I have to do all this laundry and pack all of that so they can...spray the medication. That picture is of packing. It reminds me of war in Africa where you have to pack and keep running, keep on the run.

Coding

- After organizing, or sometimes while organizing, you examine the data with a broad view, making notations of all data portions that stand out as answering your research questions and also of patterns that are emerging.

- At this point, it is crucial to recognize that quality, not quantity, is your focus. There may be some patterns that emerge because you see them numerous times and that is okay. However, there may be just one singular quote in the

FIGURE 5.5
Photovoice on Adolescents and Body Image

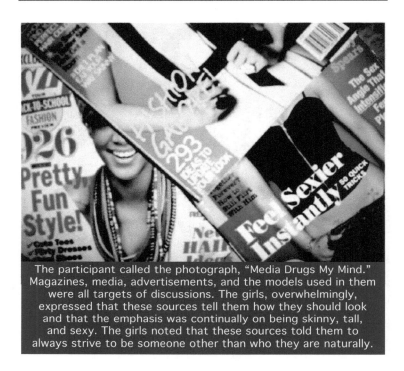

The participant called the photograph, "Media Drugs My Mind." Magazines, media, advertisements, and the models used in them were all targets of discussions. The girls, overwhelmingly, expressed that these sources tell them how they should look and that the emphasis was continually on being skinny, tall, and sexy. The girls noted that these sources told them to always strive to be someone other than who they are naturally.

narrative data that clearly answers your question and that is also okay. In fact, overlooking this type of data is a mistake in that you may be using a mindset more common with quantitative analysis in that you are thinking "more is better."

- At this stage, you may have a high number of codes that you will eventually collapse and organize into broader themes. For example, for the theme mentioned after Access to Healthy Food, initial codes may have included labels and notations such as fast food, liquor store, no fruits and vegetables, long distance to grocery store, no transportation to grocery store, eating processed foods, and grocery store closed down.

Establishment of Themes

- This is where you will group your codes into categories, or themes, that make sense. The themes will be how you organize and prepare your data for results and dissemination – these are the final story you want to tell as a result of your photovoice project. For example, in a research project around diabetes management among older black women, we categorized the photos into these themes: (a) Access to Healthy Food, (b) Access to Safe Physical Activity, and (c) Access to Affordable Physicians. All of the photos taken fit somewhere within one of these three themes.

PRESENTATION OF RESULTS

Ideal presentation of photovoice results prioritizes the main goal of photovoice as originally conceptualized by Wang and Burris (1997), which is to focus on action and reaching policymakers. As photovoice has evolved and been adapted within a wide range of social science, health, and humanities disciplines, there has been some loss or watering down of the action component (Catalani & Minkler, 2010). Therefore, we advocate for reviving this critical part of photovoice. We encourage you to plan for presentation and sharing of results to explicitly promote social action and reach policymakers during the initial stages of mapping out your photovoice project. For example, if there is a funding opportunity available and you pursue a grant for a photovoice project, then you can incorporate a specific plan for the presentation of results to reach policymakers as part of the scope of work.

As has been our mantra throughout the book, there are many different ways for presenting results in a manner oriented toward social action and reaching policymakers with no singular, "correct" way. Next, we provide a brief description of options for academic presentation of results, followed by possibilities and examples of presentation of photovoice results with the goal of advocacy and impacting social justice.

Academic Presentation of Results

Often researchers or practitioners who conduct photovoice projects end up sharing their work in academic settings such as professional conferences and peer-reviewed journals. Though this is not usually a direct way of intentionally targeting policymakers, it has the potential to eventually reach policymakers. Therefore, we recommend always keeping the goal of advocacy and policy change in the back of your mind if you are preparing to share photovoice results in academic settings. One way to achieve this is incorporating a concluding section in a presentation or manuscript that clearly spells out recommendations for policy or program changes that either came directly from your participants or are from the data generated by the participants.

A first step for compiling results is to decide whether the photos and stories should or can be shared all together in one presentation or paper or whether it may be valuable to organize them into a few different presentations or papers around divergent themes. This decision is yet another one that could be participatory in terms of exploring those questions with photovoice participants as another form of member checking. For example, you may propose the idea of presenting one portion of the data (set of photos and captions) at a conference focused on community development and another portion at a conference focused on social factors and social support, but participants feel their stories are best kept all together. It is also important to consider whether publication outlets will let you showcase the photos in conjunction with the accompanying stories or captions. For example, some journals may place limitations on the number of photos allowed in one manuscript or may charge extra fees for color photos compared with black-and-white photos.

Once you identify how to organize the data and potential venues for sharing, you then turn your attention to ensuring the photos and accompanying stories are a focal point. It can be easy to spend a lot of time talking during a presentation or writing in a manuscript about all of the process details of a photovoice project. Indeed, there may be some venues where the challenges and successes of the photovoice implementation process are the focal point of what you are sharing. However, in most cases your aim is to share the results of the project which center on the photos and accompanying stories. Design slides enhance visual display of both the photos and captions and build time into presentations to allow your audience to view the photos and narratives as opposed to rushing through that portion. Figures 5.2–5.5 illustrate approaches we have taken for sharing photovoice results in the past. Consider these images in conjunction with the process we described earlier regarding photovoice analysis to get a sense of what your final goal for analysis might look like

PRESENTATION OF RESULTS FOR SOCIAL JUSTICE

Recall that photovoice is one of many action-oriented research methods, which means that the results are *intended* to create an impact, through either advocacy, policy, or programming work that will further a social justice agenda. How this will be done best will depend on the aims of your project, the energy and focus of the research team, resources available, and what outcome makes the most sense at the time of your project's completion. The photovoice literature offers many examples of how photovoice research has been used to make concrete and impactful changes most specifically on the co-researchers themselves, including becoming change agents for environmental justice (Foster-Fishman, Nowell, Deacon, Nievar, & McCann, 2005), youth becoming voices for tobacco policy (Strack, Magill, & McDonagh, 2004), and rural breast cancer survivors of color becoming advocates for better health care (López et al., 2005) to name just a few. These examples show that the results of a photovoice project have the potential to be very powerful, bringing the visuals and words together to policymakers or even just to increase empowerment among participants themselves, and helping to create a movement toward social justice. The following case illustration details dissemination from one of our own projects.

CASE ILLUSTRATION: "REVITALIZATION OF THE Q HOUSE"

In 2008, a photovoice project commenced with community health workers setting out to examine the available supports and challenges of living with diabetes among a community of people of color who had lower incomes. The project included a statewide foundation, a local hospital, and a group of 11 community health advisors, all of whom were Black women. The women were given digital cameras to identify barriers to eating healthy and exercising in their neighborhoods of New Haven, Connecticut. The idea for conducting photovoice came from the community health advisors who themselves lived with diabetes and noticed challenges faced by their community. During the course of the research, it evolved that what the community felt they really required was a safe, community-oriented facility to get together for social and physical activities. Also, during the course of this project, there was a shooting at a local baseball field, which exacerbated the anger the community had already been feeling about a lack of support from the local government. The final action the group decided to take was to reopen a long since deserted community center called the Q House (see Figure 5.3).

After working together for 3 months, the project was concluding with the research team talking about how and where to disseminate and display the photos. Twelve photos, chosen by all co-researchers of the project, would be mounted along with the women's description of the photo on to easels and displayed in four locations of the city: (a) a senior center, (b) a housing project, (c) a library, and (d) a culminating display at the mayor's office in New Haven's city hall. A subgroup of the women attended each of these events and brought along a blank notebook for observers to react to the photos.

The city hall event drew public and media attention as well as luke-warm support from the city's mayor at the time. For years, nothing happened. Then, a new mayor was elected 5 years later. During that time, children of the women from the photovoice project had organized to reopen the Q House and presented their desire to do so with the new mayor. Funding was found, support given, and the new Q House is set to open in 2020. Many of the participants of the original photovoice project are still involved and the original project was the impetus that led to advocacy and eventually tangible social change. For more information, here are links to two newspaper articles:

1. *New Haven Independent*, October 2008

   http://www.newhavenindependent.org/archives/2008/10/when_cynthia_al.php

2. *New Haven Independent*, November 2019

   https://www.newhavenindependent.org/index.php/archives/entry/new_q_house_board/

CONCLUSION

This chapter offered guidance on ways to analyze photovoice project data for action and impact and introduced analysis approaches for photovoice data. In the end, the way a research team analyzes their project is individual. Ideally, it balances the multitude of priorities of research team members. Similarly, the overarching goal for dissemination is getting results translated into policy or programming, so working with participants as co-researchers with analysis and dissemination maximizes the possibility that the outcome of the project will be social change. Next we move on to Chapter 6, the final chapter of the book, to introduce recent evolutions and hybrid approaches of photovoice as well as emerging possibilities with social media and photovoice.

Emerging
Possibilities

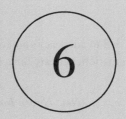

6

> *"If you don't exist in the media, for all practical purposes, you don't exist."*
> **—DANIEL SCHORR, NPR**

As we write this book, the landscape of social and digital media continues to expand and change at lightning speed, creating even more opportunities for photovoice-type, visually based research methods. Additionally, similar methods have emerged across disciplines as other ways to explore issues related to social justice and to uncover solutions for practice and advocacy for equity. Our experience and expertise thus far are with photovoice. Therefore, this final chapter offers a broad overview of digital storytelling and videovoice as possibilities that we have observed, researched, and are considering as iterations for our own photovoice work or for pairing with photovoice. We also briefly explore how to disseminate research and inspire action and advocacy through the use of social media and provide web-based resources for visually based methods.

DIGITAL STORYTELLING AND VIDEOVOICE

Similar to photovoice, digital storytelling within the academic realm is considered a community-based participatory research (CBPR) method that empowers individuals to tell their stories in compelling and visual ways. Simply put, it is the use of digital media tools to bring personal narratives to life to share digitally (Story Center, 2019). Digital stories are usually short, ranging from 2 to 10 minutes long, and elicit lived experiences of people through their own words. Just like photovoice, the focus of digital storytelling is on the story itself rather than the technology used or aspects of production of the digital format. Different from journalism, the stories are written and developed by the narrator themselves, with visuals chosen to enhance the stories (Fiddian-Green, Kim, Gubrium, Larkey, & Peterson, 2019).

Digital storytelling is commonly described as something that was developed 25 years ago outside of the academy in a community-based setting in San Francisco (Story Center, 2019). This is similar to photovoice in that both were developed as tools for promoting positive change in community-based settings, though different in that photovoice was first applied in an international context in China by Wang and Burris (1997). The original seven elements of digital storytelling set forth in the mid-1990s did not explicitly include action or change though the ethos of the method included an aim for social change (Story Center, 2019; University of Houston, 2019). Those elements are:

1. Point of View

2. A Dramatic Question

3. Emotional Content

4. The Gift of Your Voice

5. The Power of the Soundtrack

6. Economy

7. Pacing

A salient resource for more details on the step-by-step process guiding researchers in the implementation of digital storytelling is offered by Gubrium (2009). She describes her experience in using an ethnographic approach to digital storytelling that involves participants generating their own digital stories at a computer while the researchers serve as "technical advisors." Similar to photovoice, researchers lead the participant through training workshops or meetings that can be a variety of lengths, but she recommends three intensive days of 8 hours each. This is because it involves several steps such as scripting their story in a group setting to engage in collaborative dialogue, scanning digital images, audio recording voice-overs to align with the images, and learning software associated with all of those steps. In the end, the digital story consists of "voice-over, digital images and video, and soundtrack" (Gubrium, 2009, p. 189), and the story is screened for the group of participants and researchers.

Gubrium (2009) notes digital storytelling as being a forum for advocacy, which is a subtle difference from the direct listing of "action and reaching policy makers" by Wang and Burris (1997) as one of the three main goals of photovoice. Multiple professions and academic disciplines such as community-based practitioners, communication, educational research, various social sciences, and health sciences apply digital storytelling (Casteñeda, Shen, & Claros-Berlioz, 2018; Greene, Burke, & McKenna, 2018) as a tool for social change and advocacy. In one recent example from education at the high school level, Casteñeda et al. detail their experience of using digital storytelling as an approach to coalitional literacy to empower English learners and explicitly focus on marginalization and justice (2018). Other recent projects reveal an interest in better understanding connections between the convergence of photovoice and digital storytelling (Greene et al., 2018) as well as researchers and practitioners using both photovoice and digital story-telling, or components of both methods, simultaneously in the same project (Holliday, Wynne, Katz, Ford, & Barbosa-Leiker, 2018; Wright, 2015).

Videovoice is a more recent visual method that has emerged within the past decade or so and unlike digital storytelling is often described as a direct evolution of photovoice (Catalani et al. 2012; Warren, Knight, Holl, & Gupta, 2014). Sometimes referred to as participatory video, it involves the same participatory approach and principles as photovoice. However, as the name implies, the act of participants taking photos is replaced with participants taking video footage. Catalani, Findley, Matos, and Rodriguez (2009) and Catalani et al. (2012) note that unlike photovoice, videovoice is able to capture movement and audio, suggesting that it can better capture sequential narratives than photo-voice. Similar to digital storytelling, the videos produced from a vid-eovoice project have the potential for advocacy through dissemination across multiple forms of media such as theaters, television, YouTube, or other online video-sharing sites such as Vimeo. Catalani et al.'s work details the process they led in using videovoice as a means to engage participants in New Orleans in an intensive process to examine assets and needs post-Katrina and widely advocate through screening and sharing of the film that was the end product of the project (2012). Their process entailed a similar approach to what we recommended for leading photovoice, which included intensive training in the use of technology and how the method would work as well as multiple meetings to share and discuss video footage. Unlike photovoice, in this case, there was an additional component of participatory video editing that culminated in a 22-minute film that was screened by over 200 people in the community and then viewed by an additional 4,000 people online via Youtube (Catalani et al., 2012). The duration of the project was 11 months and included an 18-week training for participants. Thus far, videoevoice has been used predominantly within the health sciences (Catalani et al., 2012; Warren et al., 2014). However, as with photovoice and digital storytelling, there is a great potential for the adoption of videovoice across multiple disciplines. For example, within higher education, Giamos, Lee, Suleman, and Stuart recently used videovoice to examine the mental health of college students across five Canadian universities (2017).

This brief overview of two other visual CBPR methods is offered for consideration to help determine which type of visual method or methods might work best for the populations you work with and the goals of your research. Questions and issues to consider include time for the project, resources available, and potential outlets for disseminating the work and engaging in advocacy. In terms of time, the training stages of digital storytelling or videovoice might take longer than training participants in photography because there may be more involved with recording, editing, and producing videos. This could be beneficial in that participants gain valuable skills that could translate to economic opportunities for them, but it is also something you will need to build into the timeline of a project. Similarly, a higher level of financial and/ or human resources may be required for projects involving video. For example, the research team would need someone with technical knowledge and skill in video production. Perhaps some of the most important questions to consider and pertain to if possible, explore and decide with participants the advocacy goals of your project. If the elements of sound and music are critical in relation to telling the story of the community in the project or if the group envisions that their stories will be spread across multimedia, including social media, then videovoice or digital storytelling may be a better fit for photovoice in such scenarios.

SOCIAL MEDIA AND PHOTOVOICE

Social media did not yet exist when Wang and Burris developed photovoice over 25 years ago. However, just as Catalani et al. successfully used Youtube to widely advocate with their videovoice work (2012), there is an immense potential for marrying social media with photovoice, particularly as a means of advocating for social justice. Tools and apps are evolving every day, but some of the major options as we write include Facebook, Instagram, Snapchat, Twitter, Tumbler, and Youtube. Social media has rapidly emerged to have significant presence in major, recent movements around social justice and advocacy. Hashtags supporting social justice movements, such as #blacklivesmatter and #metoo, are all commonplace in our vernacular these days. Indeed, social media has taken on a large role in advocacy, peaceful protesting, and organizing for social justice. The public is increasingly using social media for good, as a recent Pew Research Center study shows that 34 percent of Americans have used it to further a cause or put an issue on the agenda (Anderson, Toor, Rainie, & Smith, 2018). Specifically, Blacks and Latinx express that social media has helped them to find like-minded individuals, thus helping to promote community organizing, and two-thirds of those surveyed believe social media has given voice to those previously who were voiceless, from underrepresented communities (Anderson et al., 2018).

Therefore, the use of social media platforms is becoming the next step for some photovoice researchers because of access and ease of use by populations where photovoice is often used—namely, with young people and people from underrepresented minorities. Using social media platforms as a tool for photovoice research can eliminate the process of explaining photography and ease the process of posting and discussing photos for analysis, because the use of social media inherently includes all of these steps. For example, Instagram and Snapchat are the most popular social media platforms used by young people; in fact, research shows that 76 percent of 13–17 year olds use Instagram to connect with others (NORC at the University of Chicago, 2017). Using Instagram for a photovoice project could be as easy as facilitating photo sharing within a specific hashtag wherein participants can post their photos and descriptions for discussion that can then be elaborated on when the group meets face-to-face. In a study with adolescents with Type 1 diabetes, researchers found posting pictures (on Instagram) on the lived experience of having diabetes helped participants feel like they were not alone in living with their disease, and they felt there was positive peer modeling, an increase of social support, and a decrease in loneliness (Yi-Frazier et al., 2015). For this project, a similar implementation process to what we described in Chapter 4 was used, but the first step in sharing the photos was for the youth participants to share them to their Instagram feed. The posted photos became data, and additional data were gathered through both participant interviews and the more traditional photovoice approach of engagement in a focus group, where photos were printed and discussed using the SHOWeD method.

Despite its vast potential, caution is necessary when talking about and utilizing social media with photovoice. Two major issues to consider are digital literacy of audiences and digital media ethics. Digital literacy involves the willingness and skills to use technology and must be considered for both your participants and the target audiences you hope to reach with the results of the photovoice project. This also links back to choosing between photography and video-based visual methods. If your participants are youth raised in a U.S. context who are digital natives (Prensky, 2001), it may influence your choice to utilize social media and you may have to do less training to improve digital literacy. On the contrary, if you are aiming to work with an older population from the United States or a group of immigrants from an under-resourced country who have never used a cellular phone or the Internet and incorporate photovoice with social media, then building digital literacy should be a core component of the project training. Just be sure that there is access to the appropriate language (i.e., literacy) with your co-researchers before starting any project.

As social media has the potential for reaching thousands or even millions of people through online platforms, any use of photovoice through or with social media has to include understanding and practice of digital media ethics (Ess, 2013). Examples of potential ethical problems, concerns, and questions include misrepresentation of intended photovoice photos or messages, breaching confidentiality or other ethical obligations set forth in the institutional review process, avoiding harm, and minimizing bias (American Speech-Language-Hearing Association, 2020; Purdue University Online Writing Lab, 2020). One example of risk for psychological and emotional harm that can be seen in the social media environment by even casual social media users are comments that sometimes turn racist, misogynistic, or contain other forms of discrimination and abuse. In order to eliminate this risk and other digital media ethical challenges, the ideal would be to include specific plans from the outset for how social media will be used in a photovoice project. In that case, the institutional review process can assist you in confirming you are meeting ethical obligations in the overall design for your project, and all relevant training for participant co-researchers regarding digital media ethics can be incorporated in the implementation stage.

CONCLUSION

This chapter presented alternatives to photovoice where instead of using photographs, short videos are created by co-researchers to explain their stories. Videovoice and digital storytelling allow for stories to come alive and give participants depth with how they want to present their lived experiences. Videos are a powerful tool in our current world of social media and virtual living; they communicate messages around policy change, social change, and raising awareness around social justice issues. In the end, how you conduct your study will depend on your research aims, study population, time and resources, and how your message will best need to be conveyed for appropriate social action. At the time of writing, there are profound changes in day-to-day life due to the global COVID-19 pandemic. Virtual approaches to the photovoice process offer an invaluable tool to capture experiences related to the pandemic while also adhering to the recommendations for physical distancing that may preclude in-person gathering of data for several months or more.

ONLINE RESOURCES

There are a plethora of online resources available on photovoice, videovoice, and digital storytelling. The list below is our "top ten" that we have found useful as we have honed our skills in photovoice research or as we have conducted research for this chapter related to future iterations and emerging possibilities in photovoice.

1. Photovoice.org

2. Photovoicekit.org

3. Creative Educator: **https://creativeeducator.tech4learning. com/digital-storytelling**

4. Creative Narrations: **https://www.creativenarrations.net**

5. Story Center: **www.storycenter.org**

6. How is Africa Digital Storytelling Workshop: **https://www. youtube.com/watch?v=eXPE_BnvCBk**

7. Educational Uses of Storytelling: **https://digitalstorytelling. coe.uh.edu/index.cfm**

8. The Community Toolbox: **https://ctb.ku.edu/en**

9. In Harmony Videovoice Collective of New Orleans, Part I, Introducing the Participants: **https://www.youtube.com/ watch?v=8fhok_N6sKQ&list=PLA61BF7C8034B8451**

10. Sample from In Harmony Videovoice Collective of New Orleans, Part II, Housing: **https://www.youtube.com/watch? v=eBMxrSZSCgg&list=PLA61BF7C8034B8451&index=6**

CONCLUDING THOUGHTS AND TOP 10 TIPS FOR PHOTOVOICE

Clearly, we have only scratched the surface here about all of the possible ways that the data from your photovoice projects can be used for social justice. We have attempted to provide you with instructions, tools, examples, and encouragement to confidently conduct photovoice projects. Moving forward, we encourage photovoice researchers and students to stay current and stay connected to your co-researchers to see where they think the photos should be displayed for the greatest impact. Continuously engage in reflection of these questions: "Who needs to see these photos?" "Where are those influencers most likely to see the photos?," and "With whom can we partner to get the widest spread and impact with these photos?" In the end, the power of stories shared creatively with visuals, whether through photovoice, other visually based methods, or a combination of methods, will provide a platform for giving voice to communities to advocate for equity and social justice. The Top 10 Tips for Conducting Photovoice Projects (Breny et al., 2017) are offered as a concise, final resource to summarize what we presented throughout this book for you to design a successful photovoice research project. Have fun!

Top 10 Tips for Conducting Photovoice Projects

1) It will take longer than you think: Explain the photovoice process so that you can get the understanding from participants about what they are expected to do, and to come up with the next question for photography. Patience is a virtue and will serve you well with photovoice projects.
2) Be patient about recruitment: It may take a while to get people to commit to the time needed for a photovoice project. Consider finding an agency to work with or a gatekeeper who can help access the population you want to work with.
3) Sparking dialogue: SHOWeD might work, and it might not. Consider other talking guides (PHOTO, etc.) or make up your own to see what will work to facilitate dialogue and modify to meet group needs.
4) Not about you: Don't talk, don't comment, let the speaker speak. Keep dialogue to a minimum until the presenter has had a chance to articulate thoughts.
5) Journaling options: Allowing participants to journal about their photos is incredibly helpful and may help them as they tell their story. It works for some groups; see if it will work for yours.

6) Watch privilege: Monitor how people in the group react to other people's photos. Be mindful of how one person's expression may oppress others and consider working one-on-one if the group's diversity stifles expression.

7) Anticipate that not all participants will come to every session: Include time at the start of each session to summarize previous sessions. Understand that participant lives are complicated and their absenteeism does not necessarily reflect a lack of commitment to the group.

8) Consider technology, ahead of time: Plan how you want to display and discuss the photos taken during group discussions. This also includes the type of photography equipment to use. Many people today have cameras on their phones, but not everyone has a phone, so consider how this will work in your project before you start.

9) Know when to fold them: Follow the photovoice session outline when you can but be sensitive to group dynamics. Don't force people to take on photovoice tasks if there are other more pressing issues that they are struggling with. Ultimately, allowing for time to deal with external issues will allow the group to return to the photovoice task in a more productive manner.

10) HAVE FUN! Yes, this is rigorous research, and yes, it is fun! You are expected to conduct it in a way that is rigorous and ethical, but working with photos (and videos, if you choose!) is so much fun! The participants love it and it helps them feel much more involved in the research project. You will be amazed at what is revealed when people are asked to capture their experiences in a visual way.

Source: Breny, J., Lombardi, D., Smoyer, A., & Madden, D. (2017). Getting men to explore safer sex responsibility: The use of photovoice in health promotion research. _SAGE Research Methods Cases._

References

American Speech-Language-Hearing Association. (2020). *Issues in ethics: Ethical use of social media.* Retrieved from https://www.asha.org/Practice/ethics/Ethical-Use-of-Social-Media/

Anderson, A., Toor, S., Rainie, L., & Smith, A. (2018). Activism in the social media age [PDF file]. Retrieved from https://www.pewresearch.org/internet/2018/07/11/public-attitudes-toward-political-engagement-on-social-media/

Arcus Center for Social Justice Leadership. (2020). *About Arcus Center: Our definition of social justice.* Retrieved from https://reason.kzoo.edu/csjl/about/

Baral, S. D., Poteat, T., Strömdahl, S., Wirtz, A. L., Guadamuz, T. E., & Beyrer, C. (2013). Worldwide burden of HIV in transgender women: A systematic review and meta-analysis. *The Lancet Infectious Diseases, 13*(3), 214–222.

Bonmati-Tomas, A., Malagon-Aguilera, M.D., Bosch-Farre, C., Gelabert-Vilella, S., Juvinya-Canal, D., & Garcia Gil, M. (2016). Reducing health inequities affecting immigrant women: A qualitative study of their available assets. *Globalization and Health, 12,* 2–10.

Braun, V., & Clarke, V. (2006). Using thematic analysis in psychology. *Qualitative Research in Psychology, 3*(2), 77–101.

Bredesen, J. A., & Stevens, M. S. (2013). Using photovoice methodology to give voice to the health care needs of homeless families. *American International Journal of Contemporary Research, 3*(3), 1–12.

Breny, J., Fagan, M., & Roe, K. (2016). Implementation tools, program staff, and budgets. In D. Allensworth & C. Fertman (Eds.), *Health promotion program planning, implementation, and evaluation: A practitioner's guide* (2nd ed.). San Francisco, CA: Jossey-Bass.

Breny, J. M., & Lombardi, D. C. (2017). "I don't want to be that guy walking in the feminine product aisle": A Photovoice exploration of college men's perceptions of safer sex responsibility. *Global Health Promotion, 26*(1), 6–14. doi:10.1177/1757975916679362

Breny, J. M., Lombardi, D., Smoyer, A., & Madden, D. (2017). *Getting men to explore safer sex responsibility: The use of photovoice in health promotion research.* SAGE Research Methods Cases.

Bukowski, K., & Buetow, S. (2011). Making the invisible visible: A photovoice exploration of homeless women's health and lives in central Auckland. *Social Science & Medicine*, *72*(5), 739–746.

Campbell, R., & Wasco, S. M. (2000). Feminist approaches to social science: Epistemological and methodological tenets. *American Journal of Community Psychology*, *28*(6), 773–791.

Capous-Desyllas, M., & Bromfield, N. F. (2018). Using an arts-informed, eclectic approach to photovoice data analysis. *International Journal of Qualitative Methods*, *17*, 1–14.

Carlson, E. D., Engebretson, J., & Chamberlain, R. M. (2006). Photovoice as a social process of critical consciousness. *Qualitative Health Research*, *16*(6), 836–852.

Carnahan, C. R. (2006). Photovoice: Engaging children with autism and their teachers. *TEACHING Exceptional Children*, *39*(2), 44–50.

Casteñeda, M., Shen, X., & Claros-Berlioz, E. (2018). English Learners (ELs) have stories to tell: Digital storytelling as a venue to bring justice to life. *English Journal*, 107(6), 20–25.

Castleden, H., Garvin, T., & First Nation, H. (2008). Modifying photovoice for community-based participatory indigenous research. *Social Science & Medicine*, *66*(6), 1393–1405. doi:10.1016/j.socscimed.2007.11.030

Catalani, C. E., Findley, S. E., Matos, S., & Rodriguez, R. (2009). Community health worker insights on their training and certification. *Progress in Community Health Partnerships*, *3*(3), 227–235. doi:10.1353/cpr.0.0082

Catalani, C. E. C. V., Veneziale, A., Campbell, L., Herbst, S., Butler, B., Springgate, B., & Minkler, M. (2012). Videovoice: Community assessment in post-Katrina New Orleans. *Health Promotion Practice*, *13*(1), 18–28.

Catalini, C., & Minkler, M. (2010). Photovoice: A review of the literature in health and public health. *Health Education & Behavior*, *37*(3), 424–451.

Clements-Nolle, K., Marx, R., & Katz, M. (2006). Attempted suicide among transgender persons: The influence of gender-based discrimination and victimization. *Journal of Homosexuality*, *51*(3), 53–69.

Community Toolbox. (2020). Retrieved from https://ctb.ku.edu/en

Creswell, J. W. (2015). *30 essential skills for the qualitative researcher*. Thousand Oaks, CA: SAGE.

Dassah, E., Aldersey, H. M., & Norman, K. E. (2017). Photovoice and persons with physical disabilities: A scoping review of the literature. *Qualitative Health Research*, *27*(9), 1412–1422. doi:10.1177/1049732316687731

Delgado, M. (2015). *Urban youth and photovoice: Visual ethnography in action.* New York, NY: Oxford University Press.

Denzin, N. K., & Lincoln, Y. S. (2017). *The SAGE handbook of qualitative inquiry* (5th ed.). Thousand Oaks, CA: SAGE.

Ess, C. (2013). *Digital media ethics: Digital media and society.* Cambridge, UK: Polity.

Fiddian-Green, A., Kim, S., Gubrium, A. C., Larkey, L. K., & Peterson, J. C. (2019). Restor(y)ing health: A conceptual model of the effects of digital storytelling. *Health Promotion Practice, 20*(4), 502–512.

Findholt, N. E., Michael, Y. L., & Davis, M. M. (2011). Photovoice engages rural youth in childhood obesity prevention. *Public Health Nursing (Boston, Mass.), 28*(2), 186–192. doi:10.1111/j.1525-1446.2010.00895

Fortin, R., Jackson, S. F., Maher, J., & Moravac, C. (2015). I WAS HERE: Young mothers who have experienced homelessness use photovoice and participatory qualitative analysis to demonstrate strengths and assets. *Global Health Promotion, 22*(1), 8–20.

Foster-Fishman, P., Nowell, B., Deacon, Z., Nievar, M. A., & McCann, P. (2005). Using methods that matter: The impact of reflection, dialogue, and voice. *American Journal of Community Psychology, 36*, 275–290. doi:10.1007/s10464-005-8626-y

Freire, P. (1970). *Pedagogy of the oppressed.* New York, NY: Herder & Herder.

Genoe, M. R., & Dupuis, S. L. (2013). Picturing leisure: Using photovoice to understand the experience of leisure and dementia. *Qualitative Report, 18*, 1–21.

Giamos, D., Lee, A. Y. S., Suleiman, A., Stuart, H., & Chen, S. (2017). Understanding campus culture and student coping strategies for mental health issues in five Canadian colleges and universities. *Canadian Journal of Higher Education, 47*(3), 120–135.

Gordon, E. J. (2000). When oral consent will do. *Field Methods, 12*(3), 235–238.

Greene, S., Burke, K. J., & McKenna, M. K. (2018). A review of research connecting digital storytelling, photovoice, and civic engagement. *Review of Educational Research, 88*(6), 844–878.

Greer, D. B., Hermanns, M., & Cooper, C. (2015). Making lemonade out of life's lemons: A view into the world of aging with Parkinson's disease. *Journal of Psychosocial Nursing and Mental Health Services, 53*(7), 20–23.

Guba, E. (1981). Criteria for assessing the trustworthiness of naturalistic inquiries. *Education, Communication, and Technology, 29*, 75–91.

Gubrium, A. (2009). Digital storytelling: An emergent method for health promotion research and practice. *Health Promotion Practice, 10*(2), 186–191. doi:10.1177/1524839909332600

Harris, M., & Fallot, R. D. (2001). Trauma-informed inpatient services. *New Directions in Mental Health Services*, *89*, 33–46. doi:10.1002/yd.23320018905

Hodgetts, D., Radley, A., Chamberlain, K., & Hodgetts, A. (2007). Health inequalities and homelessness: Considering material, spatial and relational dimensions. *Journal of Health Psychology*, *12*(5), 709–725.

Holliday, C. E., Wynne, M., Katz, J., Ford, C., & Barbosa-Leiker, C. (2018). A CBPR approach to finding community strengths and challenges to prevent youth suicide and substance abuse. *Journal of Transcultural Nursing*, *29*(1), 64–73.

Huberman, A. M., & Miles, M. B. (1994). Data management and analysis methods. In N. K. Denzin & Y. S. Lincoln (Eds.), *Handbook of qualitative research* (pp. 428–444). Thousand Oaks, CA: SAGE.

Hughes, T. L., & Eliason, M. (2002). Substance use and abuse in lesbian, gay, bisexual and transgender populations. *Journal of Primary Prevention*, *22*(3), 263–298.

Hussey, W. (2006). Slivers of the journey: The use of photovoice and storytelling to examine female to male transsexuals' experience of healthcare access. *Journal of Homosexuality*, *51*, 129–158.

HyperResearch. (2013). *Computer software* (Version 3.5.2). Randolph, MA: ResearchWare, Inc. Retrieved from http://www.researchware.com/

Israel, B. A., Schulz, A. J., Parker, E. A., & Becker, A. B. (1998). Review of community-based research: Assessing partnership approaches to improve public health. *Annual Review of Public Health*, *104*(19), 1615–1623. doi:10.2105/AJPH.2014.301961

Kadam, R. A. (2017). Informed consent process: A step further towards making it meaningful! *Perspectives in Clinical Research*, *8*(3), 107–112.

Keller, C., Fleury, J., Perez, A., Ainsworth, B., & Vaughan, L. (2008). Using visual methods to uncover context. *Qualitative Health Research*, *18*(3), 428–436. doi:10.1177/1049732307313615

LaDonna, K., Ghavanini, A., & Venance, S. (2015). Picturing the experience of living with myotonic dystrophy (DMI): A qualitative exploration using photovoice. *Journal of Neuroscience Nursing*, *47*, 285–295.

López, E. D. S., Eng, E., Randall-David, E., & Robinson, N. (2005). Quality-of-life concerns of African American breast cancer survivors within rural North Carolina: Blending the techniques of photovoice and grounded theory. *Qualitative Health Research*, *15*(1), 99–115. doi:10.1177/1049732304270766

Madden, D., & Breny, J. M. (2016). "How should I be?" A photovoice exploration into body image messaging for young women across ethnicities and cultures. *Health Promotion Practice*, *17*(3), 440–447. doi:10.1177/1524839915618363

Mamary, E., McCright, J., & Roe, K. (2007). Our lives: An examination of sexual health issues using photovoice by non-gay identified African American men who have sex with men. *Culture, Health & Sexuality, 9*(4), 359–370.

Martin, N., Garcia, A. C., & Leipert, B. (2010). Photovoice and its potential use in nutrition and dietetic research. *Canadian Journal of Dietetic Practice and Research: A Publication of Dietitians of Canada = Revue Canadienne de la Pratique et de la Recherche en Dietetique: Une Publication des Dietetistes du Canada, 71*(2), 93–97.

McMorrow, S., & Saksena, J. (2017). Voices and views of Congolese refugee women: A qualitative exploration to inform health promotion and reduce inequities. *Health Education & Behavior, 44*(5), 769–780.

McMorrow, S., & Smith, S. (2016). Photovoice as a participatory assessment approach for examining disparities in obesity for African American teen girls. *International Journal of Health, Wellness & Society, 6*(3), 77–85. doi:10.18848/2156-8960/CGP/v06i03/77-85

Miles, M. B., Huberman, A. M., & Saldana, J. (2020). *Qualitative data analysis: A methods sourcebook* (3rd ed.). Thousand Oaks, CA: SAGE.

Minkler, M., & Wallerstein, N. (2008). *Community-based participatory research for health* (2nd ed.). San Francisco, CA: Jossey-Bass.

Morgan, D. (2018). *Basic and advanced focus groups.* Thousand Oaks, CA: SAGE.

NORC at the University of Chicago. (2017, April 21). New survey: Snapchat and Instagram are most popular social media platforms among American teens: Black teens are the most active on social media and messaging apps. *ScienceDaily.* Retrieved from www.sciencedaily.com/releases/2017/04/170421113306.htm

NVivo. (2020). *NVivo qualitative data analysis software* (Version 12). QSR International Pty Ltd.

Nyamathi, A., & Shuler, P. (1990). Focus group interview: A research technique for informed nursing practice. *Journal of Advanced Nursing, 15*, 1281–1288.

Operario, D., Soma, T., & Underhill, K. (2008). Sex work and HIV status among transgender women: Systematic review and meta-analysis. *Journal of Acquired Immune Deficiency Syndromes, 48*(1), 97–103.

Owonikoko, T. K. (2013). Upholding the principles of autonomy, beneficence, and justice in phase I clinical trials. *The Oncologist, 18*, 242–244.

Patton, M. Q. (2015). *Qualitative research and evaluation methods* (4th ed.). Los Angeles, CA: SAGE.

Prensky, M. (2001). Digital natives, digital immigrants. *On the Horizon, 9*(5), 1–6.

Purdue University Online Writing Lab. (2020). *Media ethics*. Retrieved from https://owl.purdue.edu/owl/subject_specific_writing/journalism_and_journalis tic_writin/media_ethics.html

Rhodes, S. D., Alonzo, J., Mann, J., Simán, F. M., Garcia, M., Abraham, C., & Sun, C. J. (2015). Using photovoice, Latina transgender women identify priorities in a new immigrant-destination state. *International Journal of Transgenderism, 16*(2), 80–96. doi:10.1080/15532739.2015.1075928

Ruff, N., Smoyer, A., & Breny, J. (2019). Hope, courage, and resilience in the lives of transgender women of color. *The Qualitative Report, 24*(8), 1990–2008.

Saksena, J., & McMorrow, S. (2017). We really do have the same goals: The push and pull of one community-academic partnership to support Congolese refugee women. *Narrative Inquiry in Bioethics, 7*(1), 9–12. doi:10.1353/nib.2017.0004

Saksena, J., & McMorrow, S. (2019). Through their eyes: A photovoice and interview exploration of integration experiences of Congolese refugee women in Indianapolis. *Journal of International Migration and Integration, 21*, 529–549. doi:10.1007/s12134-019-00672-1

Sausa, L. A., Keatley, J., & Operario, D. (2007). Perceived risks and benefits of sex work among transgender women of color in San Francisco. *Archives of Sexual Behavior, 36*(6), 768–777.

Seitz, C. M., & Strack, R. W. (2016). Conducting public health photovoice projects with those who are homeless: A review of the literature. *Journal of Social Distress and Homelessness, 25*(1), 33–40. doi:10.1080/10530789.2015.1135565

Sevelius, J. M., Keatley, J., & Gutierrez-Mock, L. (2011). HIV/AIDS programming in the United States: Considerations affecting transgender women and girls. *Women's Health Issues, 21*(6), S278–S282.

Story Center. (2019). Our story; how it all began. Retrieved from https://www.storycenter.org/history

Strack, R. W., Aronson, R. E., Orsini, M. M., Seitz, M., & McCoy, R. (2018). Using photovoice to uncover campus issues and advocate change for black males. *Journal of College Student Development, 59*(4), 491–498.

Strack, R. W., Magill, C., & McDonagh, K. (2004). Engaging youth through photovoice. *Health Promotion Practice, 5*(1), 49–58.

Tolley, E. E., Ulin, P. R., Mack, N., Robinson, E. T., & Succop, S. M. (2016). *Qualitative methods in public health: A field guide for applied research*. San Francisco, CA: Wiley.

University of Houston. (2019). Educational uses of storytelling. Retrieved from https://digitalstorytelling.coe.uh.edu/page.cfm?id=27&cid=27&sublinkid=31

Wang, C., & Burris, M. A. (1994). Empowerment through photo novella: Portraits of participation. *Health Education Quarterly, 21*(2), 171–186.

Wang, C., & Burris, M. A. (1997). Photovoice: Concept, methodology, and use for participatory needs assessment. *Health Education & Behavior, 24*(3), 369–387.

Wang, C., Burris, M. A., & Ping, X. Y. (1996). Chinese village women as visual anthropologists: A participatory approach to reaching policymakers. *Social Science & Medicine, 42*(100), 1391–1400.

Wang, C. C., Morrel-Samuels, S., Hutchinson, P. M., Bell, L., & Pestrock, R. M. (2004). Flint photovoice: Community building among youths, adults, and policy-makers. *American Journal of Public Health, 94*, 911–913.

Warren, C. M., Knight, R., Holl, J. L., & Gupta, R. S. (2014). Using videovoice methods to enhance community outreach and engagement for the national children's study. *Health Promotion Practice, 15*(3), 383–394.

Wright, J. A. (2015). *Through the looking glass: A case study of photovoice and digital storytelling with fourth grade English learners* (Unpublished doctoral dissertation). Kennesaw, GA: Kennesaw State University.

Yi-Frazier, J. P., Cochrane, K., Mitrovich, C., Pascual, M., Buscaino, E., Eaton, L., & Malik, F. (2015). Using Instagram as a modified application of photovoice for storytelling and sharing in adolescents with type 1 diabetes. *Qualitative Health Research, 25*(10), 1372–1382. doi:10.1177/1049732315583282

Index